Best of Five MCQs for the Specialty Examination

T0073613

Best of Five MCQs for the European Specialty Examination in Nephrology

Edited by

Shafi Malik

Consultant Transplant Nephrologist, University Hospitals of Coventry and Warwickshire NHS Trust, UK

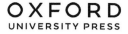
OXFORD
UNIVERSITY PRESS

OXFORD
UNIVERSITY PRESS

Great Clarendon Street, Oxford, OX2 6DP,
United Kingdom

Oxford University Press is a department of the University of Oxford.
It furthers the University's objective of excellence in research, scholarship,
and education by publishing worldwide. Oxford is a registered trade mark of
Oxford University Press in the UK and in certain other countries

Published in the United States of America by Oxford University Press
198 Madison Avenue, New York, NY 10016, United States of America

British Library Cataloguing in Publication Data
Data available

Library of Congress Control Number: 2023935576

ISBN 978–0–19–284416–3

DOI: 10.1093/oso/9780192844163.001.0001

Printed and bound by
CPI Group (UK) Ltd, Croydon, CR0 4YY

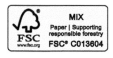

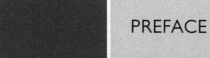

PREFACE

In February 2020, the Specialty Certificate in Nephrology and the European Certificate in Nephrology exams were combined into a single exam called the European Specialty Examination in Nephrology. There was a need for a preparatory book that addressed the standards of this new exam and I intended to fulfil that need. Given that this was a Pan European exam, I was keen to have key opinion leaders from Europe and North America to author chapters, in addition to having diversity of authors. Contents of this book mirrors the ESENeph exam blueprint and the question writing style is in keeping with the Royal College of Physicians house style. Questions have detailed answers along with further reading suggestions and at the end of every chapter, there are key take home messages. The intention behind the format of this book is not just to equip candidates with exam focused knowledge but also to upskill them by providing evidence-based answers and take home messages.

My father was a writer and I wanted to follow his footsteps, I have thoroughly enjoyed editing this book and a lot of effort has gone into writing questions. I am thankful to all the authors for their effort, not least my wonderful wife Liza, my kids Roshan and Rihaan while I was putting up with deadlines and my parents for what I am today. Thank you.

CONTENTS

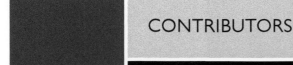

CONTRIBUTORS

Hadeel Ahmed Specialist Registrar Nephrology, University Hospitals of Leicester NHS Trust, Leicester, UK

Julia Arnold Consultant Nephrologist, Lister Hospital, Stevenage, UK

Reem Al-Jayyousi Associate Professor of Medicine, Mohammed Bin Rashid University of Medicine and Health Sciences, Dubai, UAE

Jon Barratt Consultant Nephrologist, University Hospitals of Leicester NHS Trust, Leicester, UK

Miriam Berry Consultant Nephrologist, Queen Elizabeth Hospital, Birmingham, UK

Sue Carr Consultant Nephrologist, University Hospitals of Leicester NHS Trust, Leicester, UK

Daniela Viramontes-Hörner Academic Dietician, University of Nottingham, Royal Derby Hospital Campus, Nottingham, UK

Indranil Dasgupta Consultant Nephrologist, Birmingham Heartlands Hospital, Birmingham, UK

Jorge JESÚS-SILVA Consultant Transplant Nephrologist, University Hospitals of Leicester NHS Trust, Leicester, UK

Farid Ghalli Consultant Nephrologist, University Hospitals Sussex, Brighton, UK

Rizwan Hamer Consultant Nephrologist, University Hospitals of Coventry and Warwickshire NHS Trust, UK

Mohammed Awais Hameed Consultant Nephrologist, Birmingham Heartlands Hospital, Birmingham, UK

Katherine Hull Specialist Registrar Nephrology, University Hospitals of Leicester NHS Trust, Leicester, UK

Isma Kazmi Consultant Nephrologist, St James University Hospital, Leeds, UK

Hariharan Iyer Consultant Nephrologist, London Health Sciences Center, Ontario, Canada

Gauri Shankar Jagadesh Consultant Nephrologist, Queen Elizabeth Hospital, Birmingham, UK

Saleh Kaysi Consultant Nephrologist, Brugmann University Hospital, Belgium

Rumeyza Kazancioglu Professor of Nephrology, Bezmialem Vakif University, Istanbul, Türkiye

Kateryna MacConaill Consultant Nephrologist, University Hospitals of Leicester NHS Trust, Leicester, UK

Huda Mahmoud Consultant Nephrologist, Walsall Manor Healthcare Trust, UK

Noor Mahmoud Pharmacist, Black Country Partnership Trust, UK

Shafi Malik Consultant Transplant Nephrologist, University Hospitals of Coventry and Warwickshire NHS Trust, UK

Valentin Maisons Specialist Nephrologist, University Hospital of Tours, Tours, France

Safak Mirioglu Nephrology Fellow Bezmialem Vakif University, Istanbul, Türkiye

Shingai Pepereke Specialist Registrar Nephrology, University Hospitals of Leicester NHS Trust, Leicester, UK

Javeria Peracha West Midlands Specialist Registrar Nephrology

Alexandra Riding Consultant Nephrologist, Royal Free London NHS Foundation Trust, UK

Steve Riley Consultant Nephrologist, University Hospital of Wales, Cardiff, UK

Dwarak Sampathkumar Consultant Nephrologist, Meenakshi Hospital, Thanjavur, India

Haresh Selvaskandan Specialist Registrar Nephrology, University Hospitals of Leicester NHS Trust, Leicester, UK

Murugan Sivalingam Consultant Nephrologist, Sundaram Medical Foundation, Chennai, India

ABBREVIATIONS

AA	aristolochic acid
AAN	aristolochic acid nephropathy
AAV	ANCA-associated vasculitis
AD	autosomal dominant
ADPKD	autosomal dominant polycystic kidney disease
AG	anion gap
AHS	allopurinol hypersensitivity syndrome
aHUS	atypical haemolytic uraemic syndrome
AIN	acute interstitial nephritis
AKI	acute kidney injury
AML	angiomyolipoma
APD	automated peritoneal dialysis
ANCA	Antineutrophilic cytoplasmic antibody
AVS	adrenal vein sampling
BAFF	B-cell activating factor
BMI	body mass index
BUN	blood urea nitrogen
C3GN	C3 glomerulonephritis
CAPD	continuous ambulatory peritoneal dialysis
CCPD	continuous cyclic peritoneal dialysis
CRRT	continuous renal replacement therapy
CKDu	chronic kidney disease of unknown aetiology
CRP	C-reactive protein
DAD	directed altruistic donor
DDS	dialysis disequilibrium syndrome
DI	diabetes insipidus
DRA	dialysis-related amyloidosis
DRESS	drug rash with eosinophilia and systemic symptoms
EF	ejection fraction
eGFR	estimated glomerular filtration rate
EGPA	eosinophilic granulomatosis with polyangiitis

EPS	encapsulating peritoneal sclerosis
ERT	recombinant enzyme replacement therapy
ESA	erythropoietin-stimulating agent
ESRD	end-stage renal disease
ESI	exit site infection
ESR	erythrocyte sedimentation rate
FSGS	focal segmental glomerulosclerosis
FUN	fluid urea nitrogen
GBM	glomerular basement membrane
GLA	γ-linolenic acid
GN	glomerulonephritis
GP	general practitioner
GPA	granulomatosis with polyangiitis
HD	haemodialysis
IAP	intra-abdominal pressure
IgAN	IgA nephropathy
IP	intraperitoneal
ISN/RPS	International Society of Nephrology/Renal Pathology Society
KDIGO	Kidney Disease: Improving Global Outcomes
LAC	levamisole-adulterated cocaine
LAMP	lysosome-associated membrane protein
MAHA	microangiopathic haemolytic anaemia
MBD	mineral bone disease
MCKD	medullary cystic kidney disease
MMF	mycophenolate mofetil
MN	membranous nephropathy
MPGN	membranoproliferative glomerulonephritis
MRSA	methicillin-resistant Staphylococcus aureus
MSK	medullary sponge kidney
NSTEMI	non-ST elevation myocardial infarction
OAT	organic anion transporter
PAC	plasma aldosterone concentration
PCNL	percutaneous nephrolithotomy
PD	peritoneal dialysis
PEG	polyethylene glycol
PET	pre-eclampsia
PGA	pyroglutamic metabolic acidosis
PIGN	post-infectious glomerulonephritis
PLA2R	phospholipase A2 receptor

PTE	post-transplant erythrocytosis
PTH	parathyroid hormone
PTHrP	parathyroid hormone-related peptide
RAS	renin–angiotensin system
RRF	residual renal function
RRT	renal replacement therapy
RVT	renal vein thrombosis
SCAR	severe cutaneous adverse reaction
SJS	Stevens–Johnson syndrome
SLE	systemic lupus erythematosus
Sosm	serum osmolality
SPK	simultaneous pancreas–kidney
SUN	serum urea nitrogen
TBMN	thin basement membrane nephropathy
TEN	toxic epidermal necrolysis
TIN	tubulointerstitial nephritis
TINU	tubulointerstitial nephritis and uveitis syndrome
TLS	tumour lysis syndrome
TMA	thrombotic microangiopathy
TRAS	transplant renal artery stenosis
TSC	tuberous sclerosis complex
UF	ultrafiltration
VEGF	vascular endothelial growth factor
VTE	venothromboembolic event

chapter 1

GLOMERULONEPHRITIS, TUBULOINTERSTITIAL NEPHRITIS, AND VASCULITIS

QUESTIONS

1. **A 54-year-old man is referred from the ENT clinic. He presented with recurrent ear infections. He had five courses of antibiotics over the previous 10 months for recurrent ear pain, discharge, and difficulty hearing. On questioning, he reports being more breathless on exertion and to have lost 5 kg in weight over the last few months.**

    On examination, he appeared lethargic and pale. His pulse was 92 beats/min and regular; his BP was 142/75 mmHg and his oxygen saturation was 96% on room air. His chest was clear on auscultation.

    Investigations:
c-ANCA	positive (negative at 1:20)
serum CRP	79 mg/L (<10)
white cell count	15×10^9/L (4.0–11.0)

    What is the next most appropriate management step?

    A. ANCA-specific antigen by immunoassay
    B. anti-LAMP-1 antibodies
    C. CT scan of sinuses
    D. ESR
    E. renal biopsy

Best of Five MCQs for the European Specialty Examination in Nephrology. Shafi Malik, Oxford University Press.
© Oxford University Press 2024. DOI: 10.1093/oso/9780192844163.003.0001

2. **A 32-year-old woman with a history of joint pain, weight loss, and peripheral oedema presents to the nephrology clinic. She had the following investigation results sent with her referral letter.**

Investigations:
serum sodium	143 mmol/L (137–144)
serum potassium	3.4 mmol/L (3.5–4.9)
serum creatinine	129 µmol/L (60–110)
serum albumin	29 g/L (37–49)
urine protein:creatinine ratio	420 mg/mmol (<30)

Renal biopsy showed 'spikes' on light microscopy, subepithelial and mesangial electron dense-deposits on electron microscopy, and positive staining for IgG, C3, IgA, and IgM on immunofluorescence.

Which antibody is most likely to be positive?

A. anti-PLA2R1 antibody
B. centromere-pattern ANA antibody
C. hep C antibody
D. speckled-pattern ANA antibody
E. THSD7A antibody

3. **A 55-year-old man is referred urgently to the nephrology clinic by his GP. He saw his GP 2 days ago with symptoms of lethargy. On questioning, he reported a fever on a few occasions over the last 2 months associated with general aches. He had several PCR tests to exclude COVID-19.**

Urinalysis showed blood 2+, protein 2+, leukocytes 1+, nitrites negative.

Investigations:
serum creatinine	360 µmol/L (60–110)
serum albumin	30 g/L (37–49)
serum CRP	72 mg/L (<10)

Renal biopsy showed pauci-immune necrotizing crescentic glomerulonephritis, with 58% active crescents, evidence of acute tubular injury, and moderate chronic damage.

What is the next best management step?

A. avacopan
B. IVIg
C. mycophenolate mofetil
D. plasma exchange
E. steroids and cyclophosphamide

4. **A 29-year woman known to have SLE, with a history of lupus nephritis class IV-A diagnosed on renal biopsy 5 years ago attends for routine follow-up. She has been taking optimum doses of mycophenolate mofetil, hydroxychloroquine, and calcium supplements for the last 2 years, without change in doses. She reports being well, with no new symptoms.**

    On examination, her BP was 122/65 mmHg. Examination was otherwise normal. Urinalysis showed protein 1+, having been negative for 3 months.

    Investigations:
serum creatinine	82 µmol/L (60–110)
serum albumin	39 g/L (37–49)
urine albumin:creatinine ratio	60 mg/mmol (<30)
serum complement C3	83 mg/dL (65–190)
serum complement C4	20 mg/dL (15–50)

    Renal biopsy showed 'mesangial hypercellularity with full-house immunofluorescence, including C1Q. Podocytes are well preserved'.

    What would be the most appropriate management plan?

    A. calcineurin inhibitor
    B. confirm adherence to medication
    C. cyclophosphamide
    D. IV methylprednisolone
    E. low-dose oral steroids

5. **A 49-year-old man, known to have type 2 diabetes, is found to have an active urinary sediment on routine screening in clinic. He takes sitagliptin and metformin.**

    Urinalysis showed blood 2+, protein 2+, leukocytes, nitrites negative.

    Investigations:
serum creatinine	140 µmol/L (60–110)
serum albumin	32 g/L (37–49)
serum CRP	5 mg/L (<10)
anti-hepatitis C antibody	positive
antinuclear antibodies	negative
serum complement C3	62 mg/dL (65–190)
serum complement C4	5 mg/dL (15–50)

    Renal biopsy showed a membranoproliferative pattern, with IgG- and C3-positive staining and deposits in the capillary wall and mesangium.

    Which of the following would be an indication for immunosuppression?

    A. high titre of HCV RNA
    B. presence of serum cryoglobulins
    C. HCV genotype 1
    D. extra-capillary proliferation and crescent formation
    E. nephrotic syndrome

6. **A 32-year-old woman presents at 36 weeks' gestation with severe abdominal pain over the epigastric region. This was her first pregnancy and had been uncomplicated thus far. Her BP on presentation was 178/95 mmHg. She underwent an emergency caesarean section due to fetal cardiac decelerations.**

    Investigations on the day of admission:

haemoglobin	112 g/L (130–180)
platelet count	160 × 10⁹/L (150–400)
serum alanine aminotransferase	160 U/L (5–35)
serum creatinine	95 µmol/L (60–110)

    Investigations on day 1 post-partum:

haemoglobin	100 g/L (130–180)
serum lactate dehydrogenase	2500 U/L (10–250)
serum alanine aminotransferase	1200 U/L (5–35)
platelet count	52 × 10⁹/L (150–400)

    What is the most appropriate next investigation?

    A. ADAMTS-13 activity
    B. bone marrow biopsy
    C. factor H levels
    D. haptoglobin
    E. renal biopsy

7. **A 55-year-old man, known to have granulomatosis with polyangiitis, on maintenance immunosuppression presents to the vasculitis clinic for a routine review and reports increasing shortness of breath on minimal exertion. His vasculitis was diagnosed 2 years ago when he presented with mild sinus, lung, and severe kidney involvement. He has been stable so far, with no relapses. Other than breathlessness, he does not report any other symptoms.**

    On examination, his pulse was 95 beats/min, BP 129/72 mmHg, respiratory rate 24 breaths/min, and oxygen saturation 93% on room air. His chest was clear on auscultation.

    Urinalysis showed blood 1+, protein negative.

    Investigations:

haemoglobin	14 g/L (130–180)
serum creatinine	352 µmol/L (60–110)
serum creatinine (6 months ago)	345 µmol/L (60–110)
serum CRP	9 mg/L (<10)
anti-PR3 antibodies	54 U/mL (<10)
chest X-ray	normal lung fields

    What is the most appropriate next investigation?

    A. bronchoscopy and lavage
    B. CMV PCR
    C. CT pulmonary angiography
    D. HRCT lung without contrast
    E. renal biopsy

8. **A 52-year-old man is referred to the nephrology clinic with significant oedema. He is an ex-smoker, having stopped 2 years ago when he developed angina and required a coronary angioplasty.**

   Investigations:
   urine protein:creatinine ratio   600 mg/mmol (<30)
   anti-PLA2R1 antibodies   positive

   Renal biopsy showed thickening of the glomerular basement membrane, with spikes and granular deposition of IgG and C3 along the glomerular capillary walls.

   Which immunosuppressive regimen would you recommend?

   A. Ponticelli regimen for induction followed by rituximab maintenance
   B. rituximab alone for induction and no maintenance
   C. rituximab induction and ciclosporin maintenance
   D. rituximab with ciclosporin for induction and no maintenance
   E. rituximab with tacrolimus for induction and tacrolimus maintenance

9. **A 29-year-old man presents with new-onset peripheral oedema and hypertension. He is subsequently diagnosed with nephrotic syndrome. A renal biopsy confirms minimal change disease and there are no secondary causes. He is managed with a 16-week course of tapering steroids and achieves complete remission. The patient enquires about the risk of relapse.**

   What would your response be?

   A. 100% of adult patients will have at least one relapse
   B. up to 80% of patients relapse frequently in the first 6 months after remission
   C. fewer than half of patients relapse in the first 6 months after remission
   D. relapses in adults are rare
   E. data on relapses are not available due to heterogeneity of the disease

10. **A 47-year-old woman with a past history of hypertension and metastatic cervical cancer diagnosed 4 months ago was referred to the nephrology clinic for investigation of worsening renal function. Her current medications included ramipril, doxazosin, and pembrolizumab every 3 weeks. Her next dose of pembrolizumab was due in 1 week.**

    On examination, her pulse was 72 beats/min and her BP was 138/80 mmHg.

    Urinalysis showed no blood or protein.

    Investigations:
    serum urea   19 mmol/L (2.5–7.0)
    serum creatinine   345 µmol/L (60–110)
    serum creatinine (1 month ago)   118 µmol/L (60–110)

    What is the most appropriate next step in management?

    A. ciclosporin
    B. methylprednisolone
    C. renal biopsy
    D. stop pembrolizumab
    E. stop ramipril

11. **A 75-year-old man has been referred to nephrology for investigation of abnormal renal function. He presented to his GP with a history of malaise, fever, and rash on his legs, and was treated for cellulitis with a course of flucloxacillin 2 weeks ago. He had no other relevant history.**

    Urinalysis showed blood 1+, protein 1+, leukocytes 1+.

    Investigations:
    serum urea   28 mmol/L (2.5–7.0)
    serum creatinine   320 µmol/L (60–110)
    urine protein:creatinine ratio   60 mg/mmol (<30)

    Renal biopsy showed patchy interstitial infiltrates, with early granuloma formation, interstitial oedema, and signs of tubulitis on light microscopy.

    ## What is the cellular infiltrate most likely to be predominantly composed of?

    A. Gram-positive staining cells
    B. lymphocytes and macrophages
    C. MPO-positive leukocytes
    D. neutrophils
    E. Ziehl–Neelsen-positive staining cells

12. **You have been asked to review a 38-year-old woman who was admitted with a 3-day history of fever, headache, lethargy, and reduced urine output. She has no significant past history and is on no regular medications.**

    On examination, her temperature was 38.0°C, pulse 90 beats/min, BP 160/100 mmHg, and respiratory rate 16 breaths/min. Neurological examination showed left central facial palsy. There was no nuchal rigidity or cerebellar abnormalities.

    Investigations:
    haemoglobin   71 g/L (130–180)
    platelet count   83 × 10^9/L (150–400)
    serum creatinine   279 µmol/L (60–110)
    serum lactate dehydrogenase   725 U/L (10–250)
    serum bilirubin   70 µmol/L (1–22)
    blood film   schistocytes ++, spherocytes +
    CT scan of head   normal

    ## What is the most appropriate next investigation?

    A. MRI head
    B. ADAMTS-13 activity level
    C. fibrinogen level
    D. STEC culture and serology
    E. bone marrow biopsy

13. **A 28-year-old woman who had undergone a renal transplant 3 years ago was admitted with uncontrolled hypertension and feeling generally unwell. She is currently on maintenance dose of ciclosporin. Her graft function is at baseline level and her investigations revealed thrombocytopenia, haemolytic anaemia, and acute kidney injury. A diagnosis of atypical HUS is suspected.**

    What is the main mechanism driving the pathological process in this case?

    A. deficiency of ADAMTS-13 protease
    B. disseminated intravascular coagulation
    C. dysregulation of lectin complement pathway
    D. dysregulation of the alternative complement pathway
    E. immune complex formation

14. **A 54-year-old woman presents to the eye emergency department with a 2-day history of sudden-onset painful red left eye. She reported joint aches and feeling generally unwell for a couple of weeks prior.**

    Examination of her eye demonstrated photophobia and redness closely surrounding the cornea, and on slit-lamp examination, cells and flares were seen.

    Urinalysis showed protein 1+.

    Investigations:
serum creatinine	180
serum CRP	10 mg/L (<10)
antinuclear antibodies	negative
serum complement C3	90 mg/dL (65–190)
serum complement C4	35 mg/dL (15–50)

    Renal biopsy showed interstitial oedema and infiltration of lymphocytes and plasma cells on light microscopy and negative immunofluorescence.

    What is the likely cause of her presentation?

    A. acute angle glaucoma
    B. conjunctivitis
    C. episcleritis
    D. retinal vasculitis
    E. uveitis

15. **A 27-year-old man is referred to the nephrology clinic for investigation of persistent haematoproteinuria on repeated occasions over the past 3 months. He was treated for severe tonsillitis 3 months ago and made a full recovery. He has no other past history of note.**

    On examination, his pulse was 62 beats/min and his BP was 152/74 mmHg. Physical examination was otherwise normal.

    Urinalysis showed blood 2+, protein 1+.

    Investigations:
serum creatinine	132 µmol/L (60–110)
urine protein:creatinine ratio	200 mg/mmol (<30)
hepatitis B surface antigen	negative
anti-hepatitis C antibody	negative
HIV Ag/Ab	negative

    Renal biopsy showed a mesangioproliferative pattern, with predominant C3 staining on immunofluorescence.

    Which investigation would most likely influence your management plan?

    A. ASOT titres
    B. C3 and C4 levels
    C. complement gene panel
    D. cryoglobulin levels
    E. immunoglobulins

16. **A 52-year-old woman presents with breathlessness to the emergency department. She has become progressively less well with lethargy, loss of appetite, and breathlessness over the last 3 weeks. She is found to have pulmonary oedema and an extensive purpuric rash on her lower body. She is also anuric and is commenced on haemodialysis and broad-spectrum antibiotics.**

    Investigations:
serum creatinine	720 µmol/L (60–110)
serum CRP	95 mg/L (<10)
serum complement C3	35 mg/dL (65–190)
serum complement C4	1 mg/dL (15–50)
rheumatoid factor	500 kIU/L (<30)
HCV viral load	<15 IU/mL (lower detection limit 15)
serum cryoglobulin	detected

    Renal biopsy showed diffuse moderate mesangial proliferation, numerous wire loop lesions, and hyaline thrombi in capillary lumina on light microscopy. Immunofluorescence staining was positive for IgG and IgM.

    Which of the following statements is correct?

    A. absence of fibrinoid necrosis makes cryoglobulinaemic vasculitis unlikely
    B. complement activation makes an infective cause more likely
    C. cryoglobulin is likely to consist of monoclonal IgG and monoclonal IgM
    D. cryoglobulin is likely to consist of monoclonal IgM and polyclonal IgG
    E. the presence of rheumatoid factor suggests an underlying connective tissue disorder

17. **A 61-year-old woman presents to the outpatient clinic with a new rash on her thighs and inner arms, and swelling of her hands. Initial investigations showed positive antinuclear antibody at a titre of 1:640 in a speckled pattern, positive SSA, and positive anti-polymerase III antibodies. Skin biopsies showed neutrophilic urticaria. She was commenced on high-dose prednisolone. Two weeks later, she presented feeling unwell with vomiting.**

    On examination, her pulse was 110 beats/min and regular and her BP was 185/96 mmHg.

    Investigations:

serum creatinine	520 µmol/L (60–110)
haemoglobin	8 g/L (130–180)
platelet count	82 × 10⁹/L (150–400)
serum lactate dehydrogenase	1400 U/L (10–250)
ADAMTS-13	normal

    Renal biopsy showed proliferation within the walls of the intrarenal arteries and arterioles, fibrinoid necrosis, and glomerular shrinkage.

    What would be the most appropriate treatment?

    A. captopril
    B. corticosteroids
    C. cyclophosphamide
    D. eculizumab
    E. rituximab

18. **In patients with nephrotic syndrome, which of the following glomerulonephritides would demonstrate predominantly mesangial electron-dense deposits on renal biopsy?**

    A. amyloidosis
    B. class IV lupus nephritis
    C. IgM nephropathy
    D. minimal change disease
    E. primary membranous nephropathy

19. **A 54-year-old man presents with nephrotic syndrome and severe renal impairment. A renal biopsy confirmed primary membranous nephropathy. As part of shared decision-making, you discuss induction treatment with cyclophosphamide, rituximab, or ciclosporin for 1 year and you explain potential side effects.**

    Which evidence-based information would you give the patient?

    A. complete remission is more likely with ciclosporin than with rituximab at 24 months
    B. complete remission is more likely with rituximab than with ciclosporin, but relapse rates are higher
    C. complete remission is more likely with rituximab than with ciclosporin at 24 months
    D. cyclophosphamide has superior outcomes to rituximab, but more adverse events
    E. rituximab is non-inferior to ciclosporin and achieves equivalent remission and relapse rates

20. **A 42-year-old man is investigated for nephrotic syndrome. A diagnosis of focal segmental glomerulosclerosis is made.**

    Which renal biopsy feature is associated with worse prognosis?

    A. at least one glomerulus with segmental or global glomerular capillary tuft collapse, with hypertrophy and hyperplasia of overlying epithelial cells

    B. at least one glomerulus with a segmental lesion involving the outer 25% of the tuft next to the proximal tubule, with adhesion of podocytes at the tubular lumen or neck, and without collapsing features

    C. segmental capillary lumen obliteration by extracellular matrix, with no collapsing or tip lesion

    D. presence of perihilar lesions

    E. complete podocyte foot process effacement

21. **A 56-year-old man was referred for evaluation to the nephrology clinic. He has a past history of hypertension, hypothyroidism, and obesity. He was found to have significant renal impairment associated with proteinuria, and underwent a renal biopsy.**

    Investigations:
    Immunofluorescence showed strong glomerular staining for IgG and kappa light chains, and weaker staining for C3 and lambda light chains; strong glomerular staining for IgG1 and weak staining for IgG4 were also seen. Electron microscopy revealed abundant deposition of randomly arranged rigid fibrillary material in the mesangium and along the glomerular capillary loops within the thickened glomerular basement membrane.

    What percentage of patients with this condition have an underlying infectious or malignant condition?

    A. 90%

    B. 60%

    C. 30%

    D. 10%

    E. 5%

22. **A 56-year-old man was referred for evaluation in the new patient nephrology clinic. He has long-standing hypertension, hypothyroidism, and obesity.**

    Investigations:
    serum creatinine   290 µmol/L (60–110)
    serum creatinine (12 months ago)   125 µmol/L (60–110)
    urine protein:creatinine ratio   500 mg/mmol (<30)

    Renal biopsy–immunofluorescence showed strong glomerular staining for IgG and kappa light chains, and weaker staining for C3 and lambda light chains; strong glomerular staining for IgG1 and weak staining for IgG4 were also seen. Electron microscopy revealed abundant deposition of randomly arranged rigid fibrillary material in the mesangium and along the glomerular capillary loops within the thickened glomerular basement membrane.

    What is the expected prognosis for this patient?

    A. just fewer than half of patients with this condition will progress to ESRD within 5 years
    B. nearly all patients with this condition progress to ESRD within 5 years
    C. progression to ESRD is unlikely
    D. recurrence rate following renal transplantation is more than half
    E. response to immunosuppression is good

23. **A 43-year-old man presents with haemoptysis and a history of increasing lethargy and nausea for the past 3 weeks. He has no past history of note. On workup, his anti-GBM and anti-MPO antibodies were both positive.**

    Which statement best describes the prognostic value of dual positivity of ANCA and anti-GBM?

    A. dual antibody-positive patients are more likely to relapse than patients with anti-MPO alone
    B. patients who are dual antibody-positive are less likely to relapse than patients with anti-GBM alone
    C. renal and patient survival at 12 months is better with dual positivity than with anti-GBM antibodies alone
    D. renal and patient survival at 12 months is equivalent with anti-MPO antibodies only or with anti-GBM antibodies only
    E. renal and patient survival at 12 months is inferior in patients with dual positivity than in those with anti-GBM antibodies alone

24. **A 29-year-old woman presents to her GP with joint aches and a facial rash. She reports experiencing joint pains intermittently for 3 years. Examination revealed joint synovial thickening and a malar rash over the cheeks and nasal bridge.**

    Urinalysis showed blood 2+, protein 2+.

    Investigations:
white cell count	2.9×10^9/L (4.0–11.0)
serum creatinine	110 µmol/L (60–110)
urine protein:creatinine ratio	290 mg/mmol (<30)
anti-double-stranded DNA antibodies (ELISA)	positive
serum complement C3	47 mg/dL (65–190)
serum complement C4	3 mg/dL (15–50)

    Renal biopsy reported as class IIIA lupus nephritis. The patient was started on methylprednisolone and mycophenolate mofetil induction. Despite optimal doses of immunosuppression, her proteinuria persisted and a repeat renal biopsy showed active disease.

    Which of the following medications would be effective in addition to standard of care?

    A. belimumab
    B. ciclosporin
    C. hydroxychloroquine
    D. rituximab
    E. tacrolimus

25. **A 52-year-old man was referred to the renal clinic by his GP for investigation of proteinuria detected at a routine medical check. He had a past history of ulcerative colitis, osteoporosis, and hypertension, and was taking valsartan, amlodipine, azathioprine, and alendronic acid.**

    On examination, his BMI was 34 kg/m² and his BP was 142/75 mmHg.

    Investigations:
serum creatinine	110 µmol/L (60–110)
haemoglobin A_{1c}	35 mmol/mol (20–42)
serum albumin	40 g/L (37–49)
urine protein:creatinine ratio	650 mg/mmol (<30)

    A renal biopsy was performed, which showed focal segmental glomerulosclerosis of the collapsing variant.

    Which of the following is appropriate initial management?

    A. ACE inhibitor
    B. corticosteroids
    C. SGLT2 inhibitor
    D. stop alendronate
    E. tacrolimus

26. **A 20-year-old man was seen in the nephrology clinic with a 4-week history of lower limb oedema. He had no significant past history and was on no regular medications.**

    On examination, his BP was 128/60 mmHg and he had moderate pitting oedema up to his mid shins bilaterally.

    Urinalysis showed protein 4+, blood nil.

    Investigations:
serum creatinine	76 µmol/L (60–110)
serum sodium	140 mmol/L (137–144)
serum potassium	4.6 mmol/L (3.5–4.9)
serum albumin	30 g/L (37–49)
urine protein:creatinine ratio	450 mg/mmol (<30)

    He underwent a renal biopsy.

    What is the most likely finding on renal biopsy?

    A. effacement of podocyte foot processes on electron microscopy
    B. mesangial deposits of IgA on immunofluorescence
    C. positive staining for kappa and lambda on immunofluorescence
    D. spikes of basement membrane on silver staining
    E. tubular atrophy and interstitial fibrosis

27. **A 39-year-old man is seen in the renal clinic with tiredness and lower limb swelling. He describes symptoms coming on gradually over 2–3 months. He has a past history of asthma and has a family history of type 2 diabetes. He is a smoker with a 10-pack year history and is taking a salbutamol inhaler.**

    On examination, his BP was 142/76 mmHg and he had pitting oedema up to his knees bilaterally.

    Urinalysis showed protein 3+.

    Investigations:
serum creatinine	82 µmol/L (60–110)
serum albumin	22 g/L (37–49)
urine protein:creatinine ratio	620 mg/mmol (<30)

    Renal biopsy with light microscopy revealed hypertrophic podocytes and a well-preserved interstitial compartment. Electron microscopic evaluation revealed mesangial areas of normal cellularity, with numerous electron-dense deposits in mesangial and paramesangial locations. The podocytes had extensive foot process effacement. Immunofluorescence staining showed strongly positive staining of the mesangium for IgA, C3, and kappa and lambda light chains.

    What is the most appropriate management step?

    A. dapagliflozin
    B. omega-3
    C. prednisolone
    D. ACE inhibitor
    E. warfarin

28. **A 37-year-old man who recently moved to the UK from Sri Lanka is referred by the GP for investigation of renal impairment. He was a farmer in Sri Lanka. He does not have any significant past history and is not on any medications.**

    On examination, he looked pale and his BP was 138/72 mmHg. Examination was otherwise unremarkable.

    Urinalysis showed protein 1+.

    Investigations:
serum creatinine	190 µmol/L (60–110)
serum albumin	36 g/L (37–49)
urine protein:creatinine ratio	180 mg/mmol (<30)
He underwent a renal biopsy.	

    Which of the following finding is most likely to indicate a diagnosis of CKDu?

    A. absence of casts
    B. arteriosclerosis
    C. interstitial fibrosis
    D. mesangial hypercellularity
    E. subepithelial deposits

29. **A 32-year-old woman is admitted with worsening shortness of breath presumed to be due to a lower respiratory tract infection. She complains of gradual onset of a tingling sensation in the left leg below the knee and right arm. She has had a dry cough for several months, which has been getting worse, and the GP had prescribed several inhalers, with no benefit. Her past history includes hypertension and asthma.**

    On examination, her temperature was 36.9°C, respiratory rate 24 breaths/min, and oxygen saturation on room air 93%. Examination of the chest revealed a generalized wheeze. Neurological examination showed reduced sensation in the left leg and right arm, and reflexes were intact.

    Urinalysis was negative for blood and protein.

    Investigations:
haemoglobin	12 g/L (130–180)
white cell count	10 × 10⁹/L (4.0–11.0)
eosinophil count	1.2 × 10⁹/L (0.04–0.40)
serum creatinine	95 µmol/L (60–110)
P-ANCA	positive
anti-MPO antibodies	10 U/mL (<10)
chest X-ray	hyperexpanded lung fields

    What would be the most appropriate management step?

    A. cyclophosphamide
    B. mepolizumab
    C. methotrexate
    D. prednisolone
    E. rituximab

30. **A 53-year-old woman returns for follow-up in the renal vasculitis clinic. She was originally diagnosed with ANCA-associated vasculitis with crescentic glomerulonephritis 6 years ago, and was treated with IV cyclophosphamide followed by 2 years' maintenance with azathioprine and prednisolone. She entered remission rapidly and had no relapses in the first 2 years of treatment. Her serum creatinine level at diagnosis was 140 µmol/L. On this occasion, she described joint aches and increasing lethargy. She had put this down to the beginning of the menopause.**

   Urinalysis showed blood 2+, protein 2+.

   Investigations:
serum creatinine	190 µmol/L (60–110)
white cell count	12×10^9/L (4.0–11.0)
serum CRP	80 mg/L (<10)
anti-PR3 antibodies	171 U/mL (<10)

   Renal biopsy confirms relapse of rapidly progressive glomerulonephritis.

   Which of the following would indicate that this patient is at high risk of renal relapse?

   A. ENT involvement
   B. MPO positivity at initial diagnosis
   C. renal function at diagnosis
   D. time to initial remission
   E. oral cyclophosphamide induction

1. A. ANCA-specific antigen by immunoassay.

The differential diagnosis includes granulomatosis with polyangiitis (GPA), recurrent infections, and malignancy. Renal biopsy would not be indicated, unless the patient has an active urinary sediment. ANCA against lysosome-associated membrane protein (LAMP)-2, a lesser known ANCA antigen that is expressed on the glomerular endothelium, is present in some adults with ANCA-associated vasculitis (AAV)-associated renal disease. However, the role of LAMP-1 is unclear. CT of the sinuses is helpful, along with other investigations in making a diagnosis of GPA, but the patient's symptoms are mainly ear-related. The ESR will neither support nor exclude a diagnosis of GPA, and can be raised in infection and malignancy. The initial c-ANCA positivity is likely to have been from immunofluorescence testing, which has good sensitivity, but poor specificity. International guidelines now recommend use of antigen-specific immunoassays for detection of PR3 or MPO antibodies. If this patient has a negative PR3 or MPO by immunoassay, he could still have GPA, but a positive test would be helpful in supporting a diagnosis. The gold standard is tissue biopsy where possible.

Bossuyt X, Cohen Tervaert JW, Arimura Y, et al. Revised 2017 international consensus on testing of ANCAs in granulomatosis with polyangiitis and microscopic polyangiitis. Nat Rev Rheumatol. 2017;13:683–92.

2. D. Speckled-pattern ANA antibody.

The histology is consistent with secondary membranous nephropathy and the staining is consistent with a secondary cause, likely SLE, given an almost 'full house' on immunofluorescence staining, although C1Q is not stated. Anti-PLA2R1 and THSD7A antibodies are both associated with primary membranous nephropathy. Hep C is more likely to give a membranoproliferative pattern. ANA is often detected in patients with SLE. The centromere pattern is more frequently present in patients with limited systemic sclerosis, whereas the speckled pattern is associated with SLE, mixed connective tissue disorder (CTD), and other autoimmune conditions.

Damoiseaux J, Andrade LEC, Carballo OG, et al. Clinical relevance of HEp-2 indirect immunofluorescent patterns: the International Consensus on ANA patterns (ICAP) perspective. Ann Rheum Dis. 2019;78:879–89.

3. E. Steroids and cyclophosphamide.

The latest UK British Society of Rheumatology guidelines and the EULAR/EDTA recommend induction treatment with a combination of steroids and either rituximab or cyclophosphamide. The licence for rituximab is based on 375 mg/m^2 BSA for 4 weeks. IVIg is not used for induction but could be given to a patient with recurrent infections. Avacopan is used as a steroid-sparing agent in induction protocols but is not used on its own. Plasma exchange could be indicated in patients with renal pulmonary syndrome or in those who are dialysis-dependent.

Geetha D, Jin Q, Scott J, et al. Comparisons of guidelines and recommendations on managing antineutrophil cytoplasmic antibody-associated vasculitis. Kidney Int Rep. 2018;3(5):1039–49.

4. B. Confirm adherence to medication.

The biopsy report suggests class II lupus nephritis, based on the revised 2018 International Society of Nephrology/Renal Pathology Society (ISN/RPS) nomenclature. KDIGO guidelines for treatment is to treat as per extra-renal manifestations. However, in clinical practice, if a patient develops class II lupus nephritis while already on a reasonable dose of mycophenolate mofetil, this raises concern about disease activity, and close monitoring is indicated. Confirming adherence with the patient and any barriers to adherence is an essential first step in managing patients with SLE when disease flares are suspected. As there is no indication that this patient's extra-renal disease requires change of therapy the other options are not appropriate.

Kidney Disease: Improving Global Outcomes (KDIGO) Glomerular Diseases Work Group. KDIGO 2021 clinical practice guideline for the management of glomerular diseases. Kidney Int. 2021;100(4S):S1–276.

5. D. Extra-capillary proliferation and crescent formation.

Membranoproliferative glomerulonephritis (MPGN) is a pattern of renal pathology with multiple possible causes. Differentials include viral hepatitis, haematological disorders, and autoimmune disease, as well as disease of complement dysregulation. Idiopathic MPGN is rare. Treatment of MPGN should be of the underlying cause initially. KDIGO recommends addition of immunosuppression for patients with rapidly worsening renal function or when renal biopsy confirms proliferative disease with crescent formation.

Noris M, Daina E, Remuzzi G. Membranoproliferative glomerulonephritis: no longer the same disease and may need very different treatment. Nephrol Dial Transplant. 2023 Feb 13;38(2):283–290.

6. A. ADAMTS-13 activity.

This patient developed hypertensive complications after 36 weeks of pregnancy, associated with a picture of haemolysis and proteinuria. Differential diagnosis includes pre-eclampsia, HELLP, TTP, and aHUS (pregnancy-induced). Like most patients with thrombotic microangiopathies (TMAs), it is essential to differentiate between TTP and other causes of TMA by requesting ADAMTS-13 activity before initiating treatment with plasma exchange. Renal biopsy would be challenging and will not confirm the cause of haemolysis. Factor H levels may help as part of the workup for complement dysregulation if ADAMTS-13 activity is normal. Haptoglobin levels aid in the diagnosis of haemolysis, but do not determine the underlying cause.

Saad AF, Roman J, Wyble A, Pacheco LD. Pregnancy-associated atypical hemolytic-uremic syndrome. AJP Rep. 2016;6(1):e125–8.

7. C. CT pulmonary angiography.

Patients with vasculitis are more likely to develop VTE, particularly when their disease is active. His breathlessness in the absence of raised inflammatory markers or other features of disease relapse or infection raises significant concern of a pulmonary embolus, which would be a life-threatening diagnosis in the short term and the one to rule out first. There is no indication for a renal biopsy at this point with stable renal function and urinary sediment, although persistent invisible haematuria is associated with a risk of renal relapse. HRCT can be requested later for a more detailed evaluation.

Tomasson G, Monach PA, Merkel PA. Thromboembolic disease in vasculitis. Curr Opin Rheumatol. 2009;21(1):41–6.

8. B. Rituximab alone for induction and no maintenance.

The patient's history is consistent with a diagnosis of PLA2R-positive primary membranous nephropathy. In the MENTOR trial, patients were randomized to receive either rituximab or ciclosporin at induction. Rituximab was non-inferior to ciclosporin in inducing complete or partial remission of proteinuria at 12 months and was superior in maintaining proteinuria remission up to 24 months. Patients in the rituximab group did not receive maintenance therapy but were offered further rituximab at 6 months if they did not achieve complete remission.

Fervenza FC, Appel GB, Barbour SJ, et al. Rituximab or cyclosporine in the treatment of membranous nephropathy. N Engl J Med. 2019;381(1):36–46.

9. B. Up to 80% of patients relapse frequently in the first 6 months after remission.

Relapses occur in 60–80% of adults with minimal change disease, particularly in the first 3–6 months after remission. Most often adults will have infrequent relapses, but some will become either steroid-dependent or steroid-unresponsive. These patients will require additional treatments with immunosuppressive agents.

Korbet S, Whittier WL. Management of adult minimal change disease. Clin J Am Soc Nephrol. 2019;14(6):911–13.

10. C. Renal biopsy.

This patient most likely developed acute tubulointerstitial nephritis (TIN) secondary to pembrolizumab. TIN has been increasingly recognized as an important manifestation of kidney injury associated with use of immune checkpoint inhibitors (anti-PD-1 and anti-CTLA-4). Lower baseline eGFR, proton pump inhibitor use, and combination immune checkpoint inhibitor therapy are each independently associated with an increased risk of immune checkpoint inhibitor-associated AKI. TIN was the dominant lesion in 93% of cases of immune checkpoint inhibitor-induced AKI in a recent study.

Cortazar FB, Kibbelaar ZA, Glezerman IG, et al. Immune checkpoint inhibitor-associated AKI: a multicenter study. J Am Soc Nephrol. 2020;31(2):435–46.

11. B. Lymphocytes and macrophages.

This is a classic case of tubulointerstitial nephritis. The patient had a recent course of flucloxacillin, which is a likely precipitating cause. A renal biopsy usually shows interstitial oedema and tubulitis, whereas glomeruli and vessels are distinctly normal. Interstitial infiltrates are mostly composed of lymphocytes (CD4 T cells being the most abundant type), macrophages, eosinophils, and plasma cells. Interstitial granulomas can be observed in some cases of drug-induced acute interstitial nephritis, but the possibility of sarcoidosis, tuberculosis, and some other infections must be kept in mind when they are found.

Praga M, González E. Acute interstitial nephritis. Kidney Int. 2010;77:956–61.

12. B. ADAMTS-13 activity levels.

Based on the clinical and laboratory findings, this patient has TMA. The main causes of TMA include TTP, STEC-HUS, atypical HUS, and secondary TMA. MRI head is unlikely to add to the CT findings, as neurological symptoms are caused by systemic platelet thrombus formation in the microvasculature. In this case, the patient is unlikely to have STEC-HUS as there is no history of diarrhoea. Fibrinogen levels can be requested as part of the coagulation profile to rule out disseminated intravascular coagulation but would only be useful if clotting were to be abnormal. ADAMTS-13 activity is required to differentiate between TTP and atypical HUS (TTP will be confirmed if ADAMTS-13 levels are <10%). This test should be sent as soon as possible when TMA is suspected and before plasma exchange is commenced.

Feehally J, Floege J, Tonelli M, eds. *Comprehensive Clinical Nephrology*, 6th edition. St Louis, MO: Elsevier, 2019. https://www.elsevier.com/books/comprehensive-clinical-nephrology/978-0-323-47909-7

13. D. Dysregulation of the alternative complement pathway.

Atypical HUS is caused by genetically determined dysregulation of the alternative complement pathway, resulting in overactivation of the complement system and formation of microvascular thrombi. Several genetic abnormalities in complement factors of alternative pathway have been identified, which account for about 60% of all cases. In patients with atypical HUS, uncontrolled complement activation is caused by loss-of-function variants in complement regulatory proteins or gain-of-function variants in complement activation factors.

Yoshida Y, Kato H, Ikeda Y, Nangaku M. Pathogenesis of atypical hemolytic uremic syndrome. J Atheroscler Thromb. 2019;26(2):99–110.

14. E. Uveitis.

This is a classic example of tubulointerstitial nephritis and uveitis syndrome (TINU). TINU is a multisystemic autoimmune disorder that may occur in response to various environmental triggers, including drugs and microbial pathogens. The resulting inflammation affects chiefly the ocular uvea and renal tubules, although other organs may be involved. Renal and ocular inflammation may be clinically severe and persistent, but the prognosis for the majority of patients with TINU is favourable. Ophthalmic involvement in episcleritis and conjunctivitis mainly affects the episclera and conjunctiva, with the cornea usually spared. Acute angle glaucoma presents with a severely painful red eye and haloes, with a dilated pupil not reactive to light. Retinal vasculitis is characterized mainly by inflammation of retinal vessels.

Clive DM, Vanguri VK. The syndrome of tubulointerstitial nephritis with uveitis (TINU). Am J Kidney Dis. 2018;72(1):118–28.

15. C. Complement gene panel.

The top two differential diagnoses in this case are post-infectious glomerulonephritis (PIGN) and C3 glomerulonephritis (C3GN). The key here is the time period post-infection. Almost all patients at this age would have made a full recovery of post-infectious GN, with no residual proteinuria. The persistence of urinary abnormalities in the presence of a biopsy consistent with C3GN should lead to a referral for investigation of complement pathway dysregulation. ASOT titres may still be raised but would not be sufficient at this point to exclude complement dysregulation as the underlying cause. Similarly, low C3 levels can be found in PIGN and C3GN, although the C3 level can also be normal. Monoclonal gammopathy is associated with MPGN, but staining is likely to show evidence of light chains and the patient's age makes it unlikely he will have monoclonal gammopathy. Based on the history and biopsy report, cryoglobulinaemia is unlikely.

Smith RJH, Appel GB, Blom AM, et al. C3 glomerulopathy—understanding a rare complement-driven renal disease. Nat Rev Nephrol. 2019;15:129–43.

16. D. Cryoglobulin is likely to consist of monoclonal IgM and polyclonal IgG.

The patient presents with cryoglobulinaemic vasculitis, and complement activation. There is no evidence of underlying hepatitis C, but activation of complement suggests an autoimmune disorder is possible. Type I cryoglobulin is not associated with rheumatoid factor. Types II and III are rheumatoid factor antibodies that bind to the Fc fragment of IgG. In type II, the rheumatoid factor is monoclonal, whereas in type III, it is polyclonal. Type II is associated with lymphoproliferative diseases, and both types can occur in patients with rheumatic diseases and chronic infections. Type II and III cryoglobulinaemia frequently presents as vasculitis, most commonly with recurrent lower extremity purpura, glomerulonephritis, and peripheral neuropathy. Answer C describes type I cryoglobulin. Answer B describes type II. Answer E is incorrect because rheumatoid factor can be present in patients with hepatitis C. Answer A is incorrect as skin lesions suggest vasculitis, even in the absence of fibrinoid necrosis on renal biopsy. Complement activation can occur in autoimmune conditions, as well as in infective causes of cryoglobulinaemic vasculitis.

Muchtar E, Magen H, Gertz MA. How I treat cryoglobulinemia. Blood. 2017;129(3):289–98.

17. A. Captopril.

The presentation with skin changes, positive anti-polymerase III antibodies, and deterioration of renal function on starting steroids is consistent with the development of scleroderma renal crisis. Risk factors for severe organ involvement in systemic sclerosis include steroid use and positive anti-polymerase III antibodies. Haemolysis can occur associated with hypertension. Captopril is the treatment of choice in the acute phase.

Woodworth TG, Suliman YA, Li W, et al. Scleroderma renal crisis and renal involvement in systemic sclerosis. Nat Rev Nephrol. 2016;12:678–91.

18. C. IgM nephropathy.

IgM nephropathy is diagnosed on renal biopsy in patients with active urinary sediment and/ or nephrotic syndrome, in the absence of systemic disease and in the presence of the following: dominant staining for IgM in glomeruli by immunofluorescence (the intensity of IgM staining, graded on a semi-quantitative scale, should be more than a trace; the distribution of IgM staining should include its presence in the mesangium, with or without capillary loop staining); IgA and IgG may be present, but not in equal, or in greater, intensity compared to IgM; C3 and C1q may both be present; and presence of definite mesangial deposits on electron microscopy. IgA nephropathy would also lead to mesangial electron-dense deposits, but this is not one of the options. In minimal change disease, deposits are not present, and in membranous nephropathy, deposits are subendothelial. In secondary membranous nephropathy, including class IV lupus, mesangial deposits can be seen but are not the predominant finding.

Connor TM, Aiello V, Griffith M, et al. The natural history of immunoglobulin M nephropathy in adults. Nephrol Dial Transplant. 2017;32:823–9:

19. C. Complete remission is more likely with rituximab than with ciclosporin at 24 months.

The Mentor trial compared rituximab with ciclosporin for primary membranous nephropathy. Rituximab was found to be non-inferior to ciclosporin (CyA) in inducing proteinuria remission at 12 months, and to be superior in maintaining long-term proteinuria remission up to 24 months in patients with membranous nephropathy who were at high risk of progressive disease. In addition, at 24 months, 23 patients (35%) in the rituximab group and none of the patients in the CyA group had complete remission. There were more adverse events in the CyA group than in the rituximab group. Cyclophosphamide would act more quickly than rituximab but is associated with more adverse events than rituximab. The relative efficacy of cyclophosphamide over rituximab is unproven.

Fervenza FC, Appel GB, Barbour SJ, et al.; MENTOR Investigators. Rituximab or cyclosporine in the treatment of membranous nephropathy. N Engl J Med. 2019;381(1):36–46.

Klomjit N, Zand L. Rituximab is preferable to cyclophosphamide for treatment of membranous nephropathy: commentary. Kidney360. 2021;2(11):1702–5.

20. A. At least one glomerulus with segmental or global glomerular capillary tuft collapse, with hypertrophy and hyperplasia of overlying epithelial cells.

The collapsing variant of focal segmental glomerulosclerosis is associated with the worst renal prognosis. Answer B refers to the tip variant, which has a better prognosis despite a similar initial clinical presentation.

Choi MJ. Histologic classification of FSGS: does form delineate function? Clin J Am Soc Nephrol. 2013;8(3):344–6.

21. C. 30%.

The biopsy is suggestive of fibrillary glomerulonephritis, which is a rare glomerular disease. Even rarer is the similar immunotactoid glomerulopathy (with larger, more organized fibrils). Case series suggest 30–40% of cases are associated with underlying malignancy, chronic infection, or autoimmune condition.

Nasr SH, Valeri AM, Cornell LD, et al. Fibrillary glomerulonephritis: a report of 66 cases from a single institution. Clin J Am Soc Nephrol. 2011;6(4):775–84.

22. A. Just less than half of patients with this condition will progress to ESRD within 5 years.

Fibrillary glomerulonephritis carries a poor prognosis, with reported series quoting around 40% of patients progressing to ESRD within 5 years (Mayo series). Post-transplant recurrence is quoted at around 30%. Although many patients receive immunosuppression in addition to supportive care, response is poor, with complete remission quoted in <15% of patients.

Rosenstock JL, Markowitz GS. Fibrillary glomerulonephritis: an update. Kidney Int Rep. 2019;4(7):917–22.

23. C. Renal and patient survival at 12 months is better with dual positivity than with anti-GBM antibodies alone.

The most detailed reported cohort is that of McAdoo et al. where they looked at characteristics and outcomes of patients with dual positivity of ANCA and anti-GBM antibodies and compared them to a cohort of patients with ANCA antibodies alone or anti-GBM antibodies with associated renal disease. The majority of patients who were dual antibody positive and had a renal biopsy had linear IgG, but the prognosis overall was better than in patients with anti-GBM antibodies only and worse than in patients with solitary ANCA antibodies. The relapse rate was highest in the ANCA-associated vasculitis (AAV) only group and lowest in the anti-GBM group. Patients with dual positivity had relapse rates of around 22% by 5 years. A more recent report from Scandinavia also showed dual antibody-positive patients had worse renal survival, compared to those with AAV.

McAdoo SP, Tanna A, Hrušková Z, et al. Patients double-seropositive for ANCA and anti-GBM antibodies have varied renal survival, frequency of relapse, and outcomes compared to single-seropositive patients. Kidney Int. 2017;92(3):693–702.

24. A. Belimumab.

Belimumab is a recombinant human monoclonal antibody directed against B-cell activating factor (BAFF). In a phase 3, 104-week randomized, double-blind trial, belimumab was compared to placebo, plus standard therapy (mycophenolate mofetil or cyclophosphamide–azathioprine and, in most patients, steroids). Patients who received belimumab were 1.3 times more likely to have a primary efficacy renal response and 1.5 times more likely to have a complete renal response than those who received placebo. Rates of infection were similar between groups. Based on this trial, belimumab may be added as augmentation therapy to standard mycophenolate mofetil induction therapy.

Furie R, Rovin BH, Houssiau F, et al. Two-year, randomized, controlled trial of belimumab in lupus nephritis. N Engl J Med. 2020;383(12):1117–28.

25. D. Stop alendronate.

Alendronate, interferons, and other medications are rare causes of secondary focal segmental glomerulosclerosis, often of the collapsing variant. Bisphosphonates cause podocyte injury. In approximately 50% of cases, the proteinuria may resolve after the drug is discontinued. However, renal function may not return to normal. Genetic testing in focal segmental glomerulosclerosis is usually offered to children or adults with a strong family history. The tip variant of focal segmental glomerulosclerosis is steroid-sensitive. In primary focal segmental glomerulosclerosis, an initial course of steroids at a dose of 1 mg/kg (maximum 80 mg) daily would be indicated. This type also presents as nephrotic syndrome.

Markowitz GS, Bomback AS, Perazella MA. Drug-induced glomerular disease: direct cellular injury. Clin J Am Soc Nephrol. 2015;10(7):1291–9. .

Rosenberg AZ, Kopp JB. Focal segmental glomerulosclerosis. Clin J Am Soc Nephrol. 2017;12(3):502–17.

Wooin Ahn, Andrew S. Bomback. Approach to diagnosis and management of primary glomerular diseases due to podocytopathies in adults: Core curriculum 2020. Am J Kidney Dis. 2020;75(6):955–64. Published: April 21, 2020. doi:https://doi.org/10.1053/j.ajkd.2019.12.019

26. A. Effacement of podocyte foot processes on electron microscopy.

This is most likely minimal change disease. It is characterized by a normal appearance of the glomeruli on light microscopy and immunohistology, whereas on electron microscopy, foot process effacement is often seen. In membranous nephropathy, on silver staining, projections of the glomerular basement membrane between deposits are seen in a characteristic spike-like configuration. Membranous nephropathy is uncommon below 30 years of age. IgA is likely to have haematuria on urine dipstick. Positive staining for kappa or lambda light chains on immunohistology is seen in light chain deposition disease, which can be associated with multiple myeloma. Renal function is often impaired at presentation. There is no underlying cause for tubular atrophy and interstitial fibrosis in this case.

Comprehensive Clinical Nephrology, 4th edition. Chapters 16–26. https://www.eu.elsevierhealth.com/comprehensive-clinical-nephrology-e-book-9780323081337.html

27. C. Prednisolone.

This question addresses the minimal change pattern with IgA deposits. Patients with this biopsy finding were excluded from the TESTING trial. Patients in TESTING were randomized to continuing supportive care or oral methylprednisolone after 6 months of supportive care for IgA nephropathy with proteinuria of 1 g per day. The patient in the question should therefore be treated as having minimal change disease and started on prednisolone, as per KDIGO guidelines. SGLT2i (dapagliflozin or empagliflozin) are now used as standard of care for patients with CKD with or without diabetes based on the results of EMPA-CKD and DAPA-CKD trials. Both trials demonstrated a benefit of SGLT2i in reducing proteinuria in patients with IgA nephropathy. Answer E relates to anticoagulation, which may be appropriate if the patient had a very low serum albumin level (generally lower than 20) or had membranous nephropathy as it is associated with more thrombotic events, given the risk of underlying malignancy and heavier proteinuria with this condition.

The EMPA-KIDNEY Collaborative Group; W G Herrington, N Staplin et al.; N Engl J Med. 2023 Jan 12;388(2):117–27.

Lv J, Wong MG, Hladunewich MA, et al.; TESTING Study Group. Effect of oral methylprednisolone on decline in kidney function or kidney failure in patients with IgA nephropathy: the TESTING randomized clinical trial. JAMA. 2022;327(19):1888–98.

28. C. Interstitial fibrosis.

CKDu is a new term used to describe the entity of CKD of unknown aetiology, seen particularly in patients presenting from agricultural areas in Sri Lanka and Central America. Biopsy findings are predominantly interstitial fibrosis with tubular atrophy and fibrosis. Arteriosclerosis is not marked. Prognosis can be poor, with a rapid decline in renal function. Drinking water quality and chemical exposure are risk factors.

Anand S, Montez-Rath ME, Adasooriya D, Ratnatunga N, Kambham N, Wazil A, Wijetunge S, Badurdeen Z, Ratnayake C, Karunasena N, Schensul SL, Valhos P, Haider L, Bhalla V, Levin A, Wise PH, Chertow GM, Barry M, Fire AZ, Nanayakkara N. Prospective biopsy-based Study of CKD of Unknown Etiology in Sri Lanka. Clin J Am Soc Nephrol. 2019 Feb 7;14(2):224–32. doi:10.2215/CJN.07430618. Epub 2019 Jan 18. PMID: 30659059; PMCID: PMC6390926.

Redmon JH, Levine KE, Lebov J, Harrington J, Kondash AJ. A comparative review: chronic kidney disease of unknown etiology (CKDu) research conducted in Latin America versus Asia. Environ Res. 2021;192:110270.

29. E. Rituximab.

This patient's presentation is consistent with vasculitis, and his sensory weakness is likely to be due to mononeuritis multiplex associated with vasculitis. P-ANCA and MPO are commoner in eosinophilic granulomatosis with polyangiitis (EGPA). In patients with a diagnosis of small vessel vasculitis, the classification of EGPA is based on the American College of Rheumatology 2022 guidance. The patient has airway obstruction and mononeuritis, so she scores 4 on clinical criteria, in addition to eosinophilia, giving a total score of 9, which meets the criteria for diagnosis of EGPA. It is important to note that the classification can only be used once a diagnosis is made to differentiate from other vasculitides; it is not a diagnostic tool. Treatment is based on the 2021 guidance, which for severe disease suggests corticosteroids (oral or IV) with cyclophosphamide or rituximab. In a young woman, cyclophosphamide is likely to cause infertility. Moreover, rituximab is better tolerated and the preferred option. Mepolizumab is recommended for non-severe airway disease and to minimize steroid exposure. Methotrexate can be used as induction in non-severe EGPA. Severe disease is defined by vasculitis with life- or organ-threatening manifestations (e.g. alveolar haemorrhage, glomerulonephritis, central nervous system vasculitis, mononeuritis multiplex, cardiac involvement, mesenteric ischaemia, limb/digit ischaemia).

Chung SA, Langford CA, Maz M, et al. 2021 American College of Rheumatology/Vasculitis Foundation guideline for the management of antineutrophil cytoplasmic antibody-associated vasculitis. Arthritis Rheumatol. 2021;73(8):1366–83.

Grayson PC, Ponte C, Suppiah R, et al.; DCVAS Study Group. 2022 American College of Rheumatology/European Alliance of Associations for Rheumatology classification criteria for eosinophilic granulomatosis with polyangiitis. Ann Rheum Dis. 2022;81(3):309–14.

30. C. Renal function at diagnosis.

A recent meta-analysis identified three risk factors for relapse of ANCA-associated vasculitis: anti-PR3-ANCA positivity at diagnosis, creatinine level of between 100 and 200 μmol/L, and cardiovascular involvement. Data on risk of relapse with oral versus IV cyclophosphamide are old, and newer retrospective reviews have not supported the long-held view that risk of relapse is higher with IV cyclophosphamide. However, there is no randomized controlled trial evidence to confirm this. In clinical practice, IV cyclophosphamide is preferred due to its better safety profile (lower risk of neutropenia and marrow toxicity), but concern over a higher risk of relapse remains.

King C, Druce KL, Nightingale P, et al. Predicting relapse in anti-neutrophil cytoplasmic antibody-associated vasculitis: a systematic review and meta-analysis. Rheumatol Adv Pract. 2021;5(3):rkab018. Available from: https://academic.oup.com/rheumap/article/5/3/rkab018/6164942

Take-Home Messages

1. High-quality immunoassays for PR3- and MPO-ANCAs are the preferred methods for diagnostic evaluation of patients with AAV. Renal biopsy remains the gold standard in cases where renal involvement is suspected.

2. Latest guidelines (BRS and EULAR/EDTA) recommend induction of treatment with a combination of steroids and either rituximab or cyclophosphamide for patients with AAV.

3. Clinicians should have a low threshold for investigation of VTE in patients with AAV due to increased frequency of thrombosis, especially with active disease.

4. MPGN is a pattern of renal pathology with multiple possible causes. Differentials include viral hepatitis, haematological disorders, and autoimmune diseases, as well as diseases of complement dysregulation. Treatment should be directed at the identified underlying cause and immunosuppression would be indicated only in some patients.

5. C3GN is an uncommon renal condition characterized by a mesangioproliferative pattern on renal biopsy, with predominant C3 staining on immunofluorescence.

6. ADAMTS-13 is the primary test in differentiating between TTP and atypical HUS. Low activity levels confirm a diagnosis of TTP, whereas normal activity levels will make a diagnosis of atypical HUS more likely.

7. Atypical HUS is caused by dysregulation of the alternative complement pathway, resulting in overactivation of the complement system and formation of microvascular thrombi.

8. TIN is a relatively common cause of AKI, with interstitial oedema and tubulitis being the most prominent features on renal biopsy. Common causes of TIN include infections and medications such as immune checkpoint inhibitors.

9. TINU syndrome is a multisystemic autoimmune disorder resulting in inflammation chiefly affecting the ocular uvea and renal tubules.

10. Minimal change disease is a common cause of nephrotic syndrome, with a high relapse rate in adults ranging from 60% to 80%, particularly in the first 3–6 months after remission.

11. Complement activation is a feature of several glomerulonephritides. Low C3 levels with normal C4 levels suggest alternative pathway activation. Low C3 and C4 levels are seen in classical pathway activation.

12. Management of lupus nephritis has developed significantly in the last 5 years, with evidence supporting the use of belimumab as add-on therapy to standard of care.

13. P-ANCA and anti-MPO antibodies are commoner in EGPA. Treatment depends on severity, and induction with rituximab or steroid plus cyclophosphamide is recommended for those with severe active disease.

14. Anti-PR3-ANCA positivity, lower serum creatinine levels, and cardiovascular system involvement are associated with an increased risk of relapse of AAV.

chapter 2

ACUTE KIDNEY INJURY AND ACUTE RENAL REPLACEMENT THERAPY

QUESTIONS

31. You are asked to review a 65-year-old man admitted to the ICU with a 2-day history of fever, vomiting, and dysuria. He is known to have hypertension, type 2 diabetes, and CKD stage 3. The patient became progressively unwell, requiring inotropic support and developed oliguria.

On examination, his weight was 110 kg and his BP was 90/60 mmHg; the JVP was 4 cm above the sternal angle, and he had lower limb oedema bilaterally up to the knees.

Investigations:

serum sodium	135 mmol/L (137–144)
serum potassium	6.5 mmol/L (3.5–4.9)
serum urea	18 mmol/L (2.5–7.0)
serum creatinine	360 µmol/L (60–110)
serum bicarbonate	18 mmol/L (20–28)
plasma lactate	4 mmol/L (0.6–1.8)

What is the most appropriate next step?

A. continuous venovenous haemodiafiltration effluent rate of 2750 mL/h
B. continuous venovenous haemodialysis effluent rate of 3900 mL/h
C. continuous venovenous haemofiltration effluent rate of 5500 mL/h
D. continuous venovenous haemofiltration effluent rate of 1650 mL/h
E. slow continuous ultrafiltration with an ultrafiltration rate of 300 mL/h

32. A 75-year-old woman was admitted to ITU with pneumonia and septic shock. She developed AKI stage 3, with a serum potassium level of 6 mmol/L, and had to be started on CVVHDF at 25 mL/kg/h. The patient remained hyperkalaemic at 6 mmol/L, and the CRRT dose was increased to 35 mL/kg/h. Her weight was 110 kg.

If all the CRRT fluid contained no potassium, how much more potassium would be lost in the effluent by increasing the effluent dose?

A. 10 mmol/h
B. 6.6 mmol/h
C. 8.5 mmol/h
D. 12 mmol/h
E. 15 mmol/h

Best of Five MCQs for the European Specialty Examination in Nephrology. Shafi Malik, Oxford University Press.
 DOI: 10.1093/oso/9780192844163.003.0003

33. **A 62-year-old man was admitted to the ITU for community-acquired pneumonia, respiratory failure, and septic shock. He subsequently developed anuric AKI. The nephrology service decided to initiate CVVHDF at 25 mL/kg/h by using regional citrate anticoagulation. On day 3 of CRRT, the patient was noted to have the following laboratory values.**

Investigations:

serum sodium	135 mmol/L (137–144)
serum chloride	110 mmol/L (95–107)
total serum calcium	2.60 mmol/L (2.25–2.62)
serum ionized calcium	0.975 mmol/L (1.13–1.32)
plasma lactate	3 mmol/L (0.6–1.8)
serum bicarbonate	22 mmol/L (20–28)

Which one of the following parameters would be most consistent with a diagnosis of citrate toxicity in this patient?

A. difference between total and ionized serum calcium

B. difference in post-filter ionized calcium before and after CRRT

C. elevated serum anion gap

D. ratio of total serum calcium to ionized serum calcium

E. total calcium corrected for serum albumin

34. **A 34-year-old man was brought to the emergency department following a road traffic accident resulting in abdominal trauma and multiple fractures. On arrival to the emergency department, he was hypotensive and tachycardic. His BP was 90/60 mmHg and his pulse was 102 beats/min. He was noted to have a tense, distended abdomen. Over the next few days, he was haemodynamically stable and yet became progressively oliguric.**

On examination, his abdomen was severely distended.

Investigations:

haemoglobin	70 g/L (130–180)
serum lipase	310 U/L (<160)
serum creatinine	220 µmol/L (60–110)
plasma lactate	4 mmol/L (0.6–1.8)
serum potassium	5.6 mmol/L (3.5–4.9)
serum CRP	10 mg/L (<10)

Plain CT of his abdomen showed a small retroperitoneal haematoma and massive ascites. Solid organs were unremarkable.

What is the most likely aetiology of this patient's AKI?

A. obstructive uropathy

B. abdominal compartment syndrome

C. acute tubular necrosis

D. septic shock

E. atheroembolic disease

35. **A 70-year-old man was hospitalized with septic shock, hypoxic respiratory failure, and oliguric AKI. He was started on broad-spectrum antibiotics, inotropic support, and mechanical ventilation. He was started on CVVHDF, with a blood flow of 200 mL/min, post-filter replacement fluid rate of 1250 mL/h, dialysate flow rate of 1500 mL/h, and net fluid removal rate of 250 mL/h. He weighed 100 kg.**

Investigations:

serum creatinine	540 µmol/L (60–110)
serum sodium	130 mmol/L (137–144)
serum potassium	6 mmol/L (3.5–4.9)
serum bicarbonate	12 mmol/L (20–28)

At the end of day 1, what is the delivered urea clearance provided to the patient by the current CRRT prescription?

A. 100 mL/min

B. 25 mL/min

C. 30 mL/kg/h

D. total effluent fluid rate (mL/h)

E. total effluent fluid rate × effluent urea nitrogen/blood urea nitrogen

36. **A 68-year-old woman with alcoholic liver disease was hospitalized with acute pancreatitis, septicaemia, and disseminated intravascular coagulation. She developed anuric AKI, hyperkalaemia, and metabolic acidosis refractory to fluid resuscitation and stabilization of haemodynamic parameters; she was on inotropic support.**

Investigations:

serum sodium	138 mmol/L (137–144)
serum potassium	6.3 mmol/L (3.5–4.9)
serum creatinine	520 µmol/L (60–110)
plasma lactate	6 mmol/L (0.6–1.8)

Which modality would be most appropriate for this patient?

A. CVVH with pre- and post-filter replacement fluid at 25 mL/kg/h

B. CVVHD at 40 mL/kg/h

C. CVVHDF with pre- and post-filter replacement fluid at 25 mL/kg/h

D. intermittent haemodialysis

E. any of the above

37. **A 72-year-old woman underwent colectomy for inflammatory bowel disease. Her post-operative course was complicated by Gram-negative bacteraemia and septic shock leading to AKI that necessitated CRRT. Three weeks after admission to the ICU, she remained ventilator-dependent, weak, and oedematous, with evidence of muscle wasting. She was started on enteral tube feeds.**

Investigations:

serum potassium	5.9 mmol/L (3.5–4.9)
serum creatinine	350 µmol/L (60–110)
serum albumin	25 g/L (37–49)
serum bicarbonate	19 mmol/L (20–28)

What would be the next best step to support this patient's nutrition?

A. increase calorie intake to 50 kcal/kg/day

B. increase protein intake to 2 g/kg/day

C. restrict calorie intake to 25 kcal/kg/day

D. restrict protein intake to 1 g/kg/day

E. switch to total parenteral nutrition

38. **A 68-year-old man with diabetes and obstructive sleep apnoea developed ARDS related to near drowning. This progressed to superimposed bacterial infection, severe sepsis, and septic shock. He was treated with vancomycin and piperacillin–tazobactam.**

On examination, he was euvolaemic; his BP was 102/60 mmHg and his temperature was 38°C.

Urinalysis: bland sediment, no casts or crystals.

Investigations:

serum creatinine (on admission)	80 µmol/L (60–110)
serum creatinine (2 days later)	220 µmol/L (60–110)
serum bicarbonate	14 mmol/L (20–28)
urine sodium	40 mmol (100–250)

CT angiography was negative for pulmonary embolism.

What is the most likely aetiology for the AKI?

A. acute tubular necrosis

B. concomitant use of vancomycin and Tazocin

C. contrast-induced nephropathy

D. intravascular volume depletion

E. post-infectious glomerulonephritis

39. **A 75-year-old woman was hospitalized with acute decompensated heart failure. She was known to have ischaemic cardiomyopathy, heart failure with reduced ejection fraction, and CKD stage 3 due to type 2 cardiorenal syndrome. She was taking bisoprolol, ramipril, and furosemide.**

On examination, she had pitting pedal oedema up to the knees. Her BP was 110/70 mmHg, and her JVP was 5 cm above the sternal angle; coarse breath sounds were heard bilaterally. Oxygen saturation was 98% on room air.

Investigations:
serum sodium	145 mmol/L (137–144)
serum potassium	5.8 mmol/L (3.5–4.9)
serum creatinine	380 µmol/L (60–110)
serum creatinine (baseline)	120 µmol/L (60–110)

What would be the most appropriate next step?

A. dopamine
B. furosemide infusion
C. slow continuous ultrafiltration
D. spironolactone
E. stepped diuretic therapy

40. **An 80-year-old woman was admitted to the cardiac critical care unit with a non-ST elevation myocardial infarction. She had hypertension, type 2 diabetes mellitus, hypercholesterolaemia, and CKD stage 3, and was taking perindopril, atorvastatin, furosemide, and linagliptin. Coronary revascularization was planned.**

On examination, her BP was 110/70 mmHg and her pulse was 102 beats/min and regular. Her JVP was 4 cm above the sternal angle. She had mild pedal oedema.

Investigations:
serum sodium	135 mmol/L (137–144)
serum potassium	5.4 mmol/L (3.5–4.9)
serum creatinine	220 µmol/L (60–110)

Which step would be most appropriate to reduce the risk of contrast-induced nephropathy?

A. intravenous hydration pre- and post-procedure
B. N-acetylcysteine
C. oral hydration pre- and post-procedure
D. post-procedure haemodialysis
E. stop perindopril

41. **A 70-year-old woman was admitted with poor oral intake, nausea, vomiting, and fatigue. She had a past history of breast cancer with bony metastases and was on palliative chemotherapy with gemcitabine for several months. Her medications included perindopril, atorvastatin, and indapamide. She also took ibuprofen and opioids as and when needed for pain.**

    On examination, her BP was 120/70 mmHg and her pulse was 98 beats/min. She had mild pedal oedema.

    Investigations:
serum creatinine	250 µmol/L (60–110)
serum creatinine (2 months ago)	100 µmol/L (60–110)
platelet count	40 × 10⁹/L (150–400)
haemoglobin	70 g/L (130–180)
ADAMTS-13	>10%

    Which of the following is the most likely cause of AKI?

    A. acute interstitial nephritis

    B. acute tubular necrosis

    C. atheroembolic disease

    D. metastatic cancer

    E. thrombotic microangiopathy

42. **A 65-year-old woman was brought to the emergency department with a 2-week history of nausea, vomiting, confusion, and abdominal pain. Her past history included type 2 diabetes, CKD stage 2, and hypertension. Her medications included vitamin D, furosemide, and ibuprofen.**

    On examination, her GCS was 13 and her BP was 90/70 mmHg. Neurological examination revealed hyporeflexia, but no focal neurological deficits.

    Investigations:
serum adjusted calcium	3.20 mmol/L (2.20–2.60)
serum phosphate	1.2 mmol/L (0.80–1.45)
serum urea	15 mmol/L (2.5–7.0)
serum creatinine	350 µmol/L (60–110)
plasma parathyroid hormone	1.0 pmol/L (0.9–5.4)

    What is the most likely aetiology of hypercalcaemia and AKI?

    A. primary hyperparathyroidism

    B. secondary hyperparathyroidism

    C. malignancy

    D. Paget's disease

    E. vitamin D intoxication

43. **You are asked to see a 45-year-old man recently diagnosed with non-Hodgkin's lymphoma who was admitted to hospital with oliguria. He had been scheduled to start chemotherapy.**

    On examination, his BP was 130/75 mmHg, pulse 98 beats/min, and temperature 37.4°C.

    Investigations:
serum creatinine	250 µmol/L (60–110)
serum potassium	6 mmol/L (3.5–4.9)
serum bicarbonate	19 mmol/L (20–28)
serum adjusted calcium	1.85 mmol/L (2.20–2.60)
serum urate	0.58 mmol/L (0.23–0.46)

    Prior to initiating anti-tumour therapy, which of the following would be contraindicated in this patient?

    A. allopurinol
    B. haemodialysis
    C. intravenous hydration
    D. rasburicase
    E. urinary alkalinization

44. **A 71-year-old man was seen in clinic with a 4-week history of weakness, fatigue, and worsening renal function. His past history included type 2 diabetes, hypertension, and renal artery stenting 6 months ago.**

    On examination, his BP was 135/80 mmHg and his pulse was 68 beats/min. His cardiac examination was notable for a grade 2/6 systolic murmur, and his lungs were clear. He had pale conjunctivae and 1+ lower limb oedema, and his JVP was 3 cm above the sternal angle.

    Urinalysis showed protein trace.

    Investigations:
haemoglobin	98 g/L (130–180)
serum creatinine	380 µmol/L (60–110)
serum adjusted calcium	2.7 mmol/L (2.20–2.60)
serum albumin	38 g/L (37–49)
plasma parathyroid hormone	0.5 pmol/L (09–5.4)
urine protein:creatinine ratio	200 mg/mmol (<30)

    Doppler ultrasound of the kidneys demonstrated good flow.

    What is the renal biopsy likely to show?

    A. diabetic nephropathy
    B. hypertensive nephrosclerosis
    C. light chain deposition disease
    D. pauci-immune glomerulonephritis
    E. renal infarction

45. **A 65-year-old-man presented to the emergency department with a 6-week history of painless gross haematuria and weakness. He was diagnosed with renal cell carcinoma, for which he underwent laparoscopic left nephrectomy and chemotherapy with bevacizumab. Four weeks after starting treatment, he was noted to have hypertension. He was taking furosemide, metoprolol, amlodipine, and ibuprofen occasionally. Over the next 4 days, his renal function declines rapidly.**

Investigations
serum creatinine   400 µmol/L (60–110)
serum creatinine (on admission)   110 µmol/L (60–110)
platelet count   80 × 10⁹/L (150–400)
haemoglobin   99 g/L (130–180)
white cell count   8.8 × 10⁹/L (4.0–11.0)
Renal biopsy report is awaited.

What is the biopsy likely to show?

A. acute interstitial nephritis
B. acute tubular necrosis
C. necrotizing vasculitis
D. onion skinning from hypertensive nephropathy
E. thrombotic microangiopathy

46. **A 72-year-old woman was admitted with weight loss, fatigue, and fever. She had a history of triple-negative breast cancer, hypertension, atrial fibrillation, and chronic low back pain. Six weeks earlier, she was diagnosed with non-resectable metastatic disease with retroperitoneal and intrathoracic lymphadenopathy. She was taking metoprolol, warfarin, pembrolizumab, aciclovir, and acetaminophen.**

On examination, her BP was 150/85 mmHg and she had mild lower limb oedema. Urinalysis showed specific gravity 1.010, protein trace, blood 1+.

Investigations:
serum creatinine   300 µmol/L (60–110)
serum albumin   40 g/L (37–49)
white cell count   13.5 (4.0–11.0)
eosinonhil count   1.5 (0.04–0.40)

What is the most likely cause for the AKI?

A. acute interstitial nephritis
B. acute tubular necrosis
C. crystal-induced nephropathy
D. necrotizing glomerulonephritis
E. thrombotic microangiopathy

47. **A 52-year-old woman presented to the emergency department with a 2-week history of worsening leg swelling, gross haematuria, reduced urine output, and lower extremity skin rash. She was known to have hypertension and hepatitis C infection, and was HIV-positive. She admitted to intermittently using cocaine. She had completed treatment for hepatitis C infection and achieved sustained viral remission. She was taking losartan, multivitamins, naproxen, and herbal products.**

On examination, she had conjunctival pallor, petechial non-blanching skin lesions on both shins, and pitting lower limb oedema. Her BP was 164/98 mmHg and her pulse was 102 beats/min. On chest examination, there were bibasal lung crepitations.

Urinalysis showed protein 2+, blood 2+.

Investigations:
platelet count	150 × 10⁹/L (150–400)
serum creatinine	360 μmol/L (60–110)
serum albumin	38 g/L (37–49)
urine protein:creatinine ratio	40 mg/mmol (<30)
serum haptoglobin	1 g/L (0.13–1.63)

Chest X-ray showed bilateral coarse lung opacities.
A renal biopsy was obtained.

What histological lesion is likely to be seen on the biopsy?

A. membranoproliferative glomerulonephritis
B. membranous nephropathy
C. minimal change disease
D. necrotizing glomerulonephritis with crescents
E. thrombotic microangiopathy

48. **A 74-year-old man underwent open reduction and internal fixation of a hip fracture. He was given 2 units of blood transfusion and 3 L of hydroxyethyl starch intra- and perioperatively for volume expansion and haemodynamic support. Post-operatively, he was treated with IV vancomycin for *Staphylococcus aureus* bacteraemia. His past history included hypertension, hyperlipidaemia, CKD stage 3, and coronary artery disease. He was taking ramipril, bisoprolol, and atorvastatin.**

    On examination, his BP was 118/70 mmHg and his pulse was 100 beats/min; his JVP was 6 cm above the sternal angle. He had mild pedal oedema and bibasal crepitations. Over the next 72 hours, he developed oliguria resistant to high-dose IV furosemide.

    Urine dipstick showed specific gravity 1.010, pH 5.5, protein 1+.

    Investigations:
    serum creatinine   390 µmol/L (60–110)
    serum creatinine (4 months ago)   150 µmol/L (60–110)
    serum albumin   38 g/L (37–49)
    white cell count   13.5 × 10^9/L (4.0–11.0)

    Renal biopsy showed swelling and vacuolization of renal tubular cells.

    What is the likely cause of the AKI?

    A. high-dose furosemide
    B. hydroxyethyl starch
    C. ramipril
    D. septicaemia
    E. vancomycin-induced nephrotoxicity

49. **A 50-year-old woman presented to the emergency department 4 hours after taking 100 pills of aspirin 325 mg each. Her past history included depression, previous suicidal attempts, and osteoarthritis, and she was taking escitalopram and tramadol. She was given activated charcoal and vomited shortly after arrival.**

    On examination, her GCS was 15, BP 160/90 mmHg, pulse 86 beats/min and regular, and respiratory rate 30 breaths/min. There was mild epigastric tenderness.

    Investigations:
    serum sodium   135 mmol/L (137–144)
    serum potassium   4.3 mmol/L (3.5–4.9)
    serum creatinine   100 µmol/L (60–110)
    salicylate level   5 mmol/L (1.1–2.2 mmol/L)
    serum creatinine   100 µmol/L (60–110)
    Arterial blood gas pH   7.46 (7.35–7.45)
    bicarbonate   17 mmol/L (21–29)
    Pco_2 2.5 kPa (4.7–6.0)
    Po_2 (on 2L oxygen)   13 kPa (11.3–12.6)

    What is the next best management step?

    A. activated charcoal

B. continuous renal replacement therapy

C. fluids and furosemide

D. haemodialysis

E. urinary alkalinization

50. **A 50-year-old woman was seen in the bariatric surgery clinic for consideration of weight reduction surgery. She had a past history of hypertension, osteoarthritis, type 2 diabetes, and morbid obesity. She reported feeling tired and exhausted for 2–3 weeks. She was taking irbesartan, linagliptin, ibuprofen, and a health store weight loss supplement for the past 3 years.**

On examination, her BMI was 40 kg/m² and her BP was 160/92 mmHg; there was no pedal oedema.

Urinalysis showed protein trace, glucose 2+.

Investigations:
serum creatinine 280 µmol/L (60–110)
serum albumin 36 g/L (37–49)

Renal biopsy showed extensive interstitial fibrosis, tubular atrophy, and shrunken glomeruli. Immunofluorescence was negative, and no electron-dense deposits were seen on electron microscopy.

What is the most likely explanation for the renal impairment?

A. aristolochic acid nephropathy

B. diabetic nephropathy

C. interstitial nephritis

D. acute tubular injury

E. secondary FSGS

31. A. Continuous venovenous haemodiafiltration effluent rate of 2750 mL/h.

Option A is the only one that provides the recommended minimum dose of CRRT of 20–25 mL/kg/h (total effluent rate of 2750 mL/h divided by the patient's weight of 110 kg = 25 mL/kg/h). Option D is incorrect, as it provides an inadequate dose of CRRT (15 mL/kg/h). Options B (35 mL/kg/h) and C (50 mL/kg/h) are incorrect, as they provide higher doses than necessary. In the RENAL study, there was no difference in mortality rates between CVVHDF at 25 mL/kg/h and CVVHDG at 40 mL/kg/h. Slow continuous ultrafiltration will not provide solute clearance.

RENAL Replacement Therapy Study Investigators; Bellomo R, Cass A, Cole L, Finfer S, Gallagher M, Lo S, McArthur C, McGuinness S, Myburgh J, Norton R, Scheinkestel C, Su S. Intensity of continuous renal-replacement therapy in critically ill patients. N Engl J Med. 2009 Oct 22;361(17):1627–38. doi:10.1056/NEJMoa0902413.

Palevsky PM, O'Connor TZ, Chertow GM, Crowley ST, Zhang JH, Kellum JA; US Department of Veterans Affairs/National Institutes of Health Acute Renal Failure Trial Network. Intensity of renal replacement therapy in acute kidney injury: perspective from within the Acute Renal Failure Trial Network Study. Crit Care. 2009;13(4):310.

32. B. 6.6 mmol/h.

Initial prescribed dose was 25 mL/kg/h = 2.750 L/h (25 mL/h × 110 kg = 2750). Potassium lost in the effluent = 6 mmol/L × 2.75 L/h = 16.5 mmol/h.

Prescribed dose was increased to 35 mL/kg/h = 3.85 L/h (35 mL/h × 110 kg = 3850). Potassium lost in the effluent = 6 mmol/L × 3.85 L/h = 23.1 mmol/h.

Therefore, when the dose of CVVHDF was increased to 35 mL/kg/h, potassium removal would increase by 6.6 mmol/h (23.1 mmol/h − 16.5 mmol/h = 6.6 mmol/h).

Neyra JA, Tolwani A. CRRT prescription and delivery of dose. Semin Dial. 2021;34(6):432–9.

33. D. Ratio of total serum calcium to ionized serum calcium.

Citrate chelates free calcium in the extracorporeal circuit and prevents activation of the calcium-dependent coagulation pathway. Post-filter ionized calcium is used to measure the anticoagulant effect of citrate, and total serum calcium is used to determine the rate of calcium infusion. Risk factors for citrate toxicity include liver disease, lactic acidosis, and hypoperfusion at a cellular level. Findings of citrate toxicity include worsening metabolic acidosis, increasing calcium infusion requirements, and decreasing systemic ionized calcium and calcium ratio (total calcium:ionized calcium ratio) (also referred to as calcium gap) of >2.5:1. In this example, the ratio is 2.6/0.975 = 2.66. Option A is incorrect, as the difference between total and ionized calcium is not a validated tool to diagnose citrate toxicity. Option C is incorrect, as an elevated anion gap by itself is not sufficient to diagnose citrate toxicity and could be due to a variety of other factors (ongoing sepsis, hyperlactataemia, etc.).

Meier-Kriesche HU, Gitomer J, Finkel K, DuBose T. Increased total to ionized calcium ratio during continuous venovenous hemodialysis with regional citrate anticoagulation. Crit Care Med. 2001 Apr;29(4):748–52.

34. B. Abdominal compartment syndrome.

This patient has features consistent with abdominal compartment syndrome: blunt abdominal trauma, haemodynamic instability, intra-abdominal bleeding, and massive abdominal distension. Diagnosis can be made by indirect measurement of intra-abdominal pressure with an intravesicular catheter (e.g. Foley catheter). Increased intra-abdominal pressure (IAP) has an impact on multiple organ systems: decreased cardiac output and venous return, decreased splanchnic perfusion, increased intrathoracic and airway pressures, decreased intracranial perfusion pressure, and decreased renal perfusion. The latter leads to decreased GFR and urine output. The following grading system is used to categorize abdominal compartment syndrome:

Grade I: IAP 12–15 mmHg (intra-abdominal hypertension)

Grade II: IAP 16–20 mmHg

Grade III: IAP 21–25 mmHg

Grade IV: IAP >25 mmHg.

Options A, C, D, and E are incorrect, as there are no clinical or radiological features pointing towards obstruction, ongoing septic shock, or an atheroembolic phenomenon. Although acute tubular necrosis could be a possibility, it is not most likely, given all the other features.

Vatankhah S, Sheikhi RA, Heidari M, Moradimajd P. The relationship between fluid resuscitation and intra-abdominal hypertension in patients with blunt abdominal trauma. Int J Crit Illn Inj Sci. 2018 Jul-Sep;8(3):149–53.

35. E. Total effluent fluid rate × effluent urea nitrogen/blood urea nitrogen.

Prescribed dose is 30 mL/kg/h (prescribed dose = total effluent fluid rate/body weight = 1250 + 1500 + 250 = 3000/100 = 30 mL/kg/h) (Option C). However, the delivered dose is often less than the prescribed dose. This is because filter permeability and efficacy decline over time due to concentration polarization (concentration of rejected solvents on the membrane surface), protein fouling, and filter clotting. Additionally, downtime occurring as a result of investigations (CT scan, MRI, etc.) must be taken into account. At any given time, the sieving properties of the membrane can be estimated by measuring the effluent fluid urea nitrogen (FUN):blood urea nitrogen (BUN) ratio. Delivered dose = total effluent fluid rate × FUN/BUN (Option E, which is the correct answer). The decline in the FUN/BUN ratio is associated with a significant difference between the prescribed and the delivered clearance of small solutes. Option D is incorrect, as the effluent rate must be adjusted for body weight.

Granado RC, Macedo E, Chertow GM, et al. Effluent volume in continuous renal replacement therapy overestimates the delivered dose of dialysis. Clin J Am Soc Nephrol. 2011;6:467–75.

Macedo E, Claure-Del Granado R, Mehta RL. Effluent volume and dialysis dose in CRRT: time for reappraisal. Nat Rev Nephrol. 2011 Nov 1;8(1):57–60.

36. E. Any of the above.

Studies have shown no overall benefit on outcomes of CRRT, compared to intermittent haemodialysis. The ATN trial compared intermittent haemodialysis vs CVVHDF vs SLED at intensive and less intensive doses, and found no difference on mortality or renal recovery. Although convective therapies such as haemofiltration may increase medium to large molecule clearance, they may also shorten filter life. Also, no CRRT modality has been shown to be superior. The choice of modality depends on local practice and expertise, resource availability, and one with the least likelihood for errors. There is also no benefit of intensive/high-dose therapy over conventional CRRT on patient survival, renal function recovery, and cytokine removal in critically ill patients with AKI (HICORES trial). With CRRT, an effluent flow rate of at least 20 mL/kg/h should be targeted. Careful attention should be paid to ensure that this target dose is delivered (accommodating for filter downtime, declining membrane efficacy over time, etc.).

Friedrich JO, Wald R, Bagshaw SM, et al. Hemofiltration compared to hemodialysis for acute kidney injury: systematic review and meta-analysis. Crit Care. 2012 Aug 6;16(4):R146.

VA/NIH Acute Renal Failure Trial Network; Palevsky PM, Zhang JH, O'Connor TZ, et al. Intensity of renal support in critically ill patients with acute kidney injury. N Engl J Med. 2008 Jul 3;359(1):7–20.

Park JT, Lee H, Kee YK, et al. HICORES Investigators. High-dose versus conventional-dose continuous venovenous hemodiafiltration and patient and kidney survival and cytokine removal in sepsis-associated acute kidney injury: a randomized controlled trial. Am J Kidney Dis. 2016 Oct;68(4):599–608.

37. B. Increase protein intake to 2 g/kg/day.

Malnutrition is very common in critically ill patients. Critical illness is a hypermetabolic state, and energy demands are often met by muscle proteolysis. Thirty to 50% of ICU patients have evidence of protein–energy malnutrition. Through non-selective clearance and promotion of a negative nitrogen balance, CRRT accelerates nutritional losses and contributes to protein malnutrition. It also augments the loss of trace elements, micronutrients, and water-soluble vitamins. Low serum albumin and pre-albumin levels are indicators of poor nutritional status. Hypophosphataemia during CRRT is associated with prolonged respiratory failure. Although CRRT prescription impacts nutritional needs, with higher doses resulting in more nutritional losses, total caloric needs generally remain unchanged (Option A is incorrect). Enteral nutrition is safe and more practical than, and superior to, parenteral nutrition (Option E is incorrect). Protein restriction is not recommended in AKI, especially in the ICU (Option D is incorrect). In fact, daily protein intake should be increased to 1.5–2.5 g/kg/day to reach a positive nitrogen balance (Option B, which is the correct answer).

Gervasio JM, Garmon WP, Holowatyj M. Nutrition support in acute kidney injury. Nutr Clin Pract. 2011 Aug;26(4):374–81.

McClave SA, Taylor BE, Martindale RG, et al. Society of Critical Care Medicine; American Society for Parenteral and Enteral Nutrition. Guidelines for the Provision and Assessment of Nutrition Support Therapy in the Adult Critically Ill Patient: Society of Critical Care Medicine (SCCM) and American Society for Parenteral and Enteral Nutrition (A.S.P.E.N.). JPEN J Parenter Enteral Nutr. 2016 Feb;40(2):159–211.

Demirjian S, Teo BW, Guzman JA, et al. Hypophosphatemia during continuous hemodialysis is associated with prolonged respiratory failure in patients with acute kidney injury. Nephrol Dial Transplant. 2011 Nov;26(11):3508–14.

38. B. Concomitant use of vancomycin and Tazocin

Several cohort studies, systematic reviews, and meta-analyses have shown an association between piperacillin–tazobactam and vancomycin combination therapy and an increased incidence of AKI. Risk factors include high trough vancomycin levels, concurrent treatment with nephrotoxic agents, CKD, prolonged duration of therapy, obesity, and critically illness. Although the pathogenesis has not been clearly defined, there may be a synergistic phenomenon since piperacillin–tazobactam alone has negligible nephrotoxicity. Proposed mechanisms include decreased clearance of vancomycin by piperacillin leading to bioaccumulation, induction of subclinical interstitial nephritis by beta-lactam agents, and direct tubular toxicity associated with vancomycin. Piperacillin exposure inhibits organic anion transporters (OAT 1 and 3), whereas vancomycin may reduce the cellular expression of these transporters, decreasing the tubular secretion of creatinine. There is no clinical evidence of volume depletion (Option A is incorrect). The timeline of AKI does not fit with acute tubular necrosis or contrast-induced nephropathy. There are no features to suggest post-infectious glomerulonephritis.

Blair M, Côté JM, Cotter A, et al. Nephrotoxicity from Vancomycin Combined with Piperacillin-Tazobactam: A Comprehensive Review. Am J Nephrol. 2021;52(2):85–97.

Elyasi S, Khalili H. Vancomycin dosing nomograms targeting high serum trough levels in different populations: pros and cons. Eur J Clin Pharmacol. 2016 Jul;72(7):777–88.

Gomes DM, Smotherman C, Birch A, et al. Comparison of acute kidney injury during treatment with vancomycin in combination with piperacillin-tazobactam or cefepime. Pharmacotherapy. 2014 Jul;34(7):662–9.

Hammond DA, Smith MN, Li C, et al. Systematic review and meta-analysis of acute kidney injury associated with concomitant vancomycin and piperacillin/tazobactam. Clin Infect Dis. 2017 Mar 1;64(5):666–74.

39. E. Stepped diuretic therapy.

Low-dose dopamine has been found to be harmful by worsening renal perfusion and increasing renal resistive indices in patients with AKI. The CARRESS-HF study was a randomized trial that compared the impact of stepped diuretic therapy vs ultrafiltration on volume removal, weight loss, and preservation of renal function in hospitalized patients with acute decompensated heart failure and cardiorenal syndrome. Stepped pharmacological therapy was found to be superior to ultrafiltration for preservation of renal function at 96 hours, with a similar amount of weight loss. Ultrafiltration was associated with a higher rate of adverse events. Stepped pharmacological care includes titrating the dose of loop diuretics (increasing or decreasing the dose, or continuing the current dose) and/or adding a thiazide diuretic (such as metolazone) to maintain a urine output of 3–5 L/day. Addition of spironolactone would increase the risk of worsening hyperkalaemia and would not be sufficient to manage volume overload and AKI.

Bart BA, Goldsmith SR, Lee KL, et al. CARRESS-HF. Ultrafiltration in decompensated heart failure with cardiorenal syndrome. N Engl J Med. 2012;367:2296–304.

40. A. Intravenous hydration pre- and post-procedure.

The PRESERVE trial found no benefit of peri-procedural IV isotonic sodium bicarbonate over IV isotonic sodium chloride with respect to the risk of major adverse kidney events, death, or AKI in patients with impaired renal function undergoing angiography. In addition, there was no benefit of oral administration of acetylcysteine over placebo in decreasing the same risks. The 2012 KDIGO Clinical Practice Guidelines recommend using volume expansion with either isotonic sodium chloride or sodium bicarbonate in patients at risk of contrast-induced nephropathy. N-acetylcysteine is best used concurrently with IV isotonic crystalloids, not in isolation. Withholding ACE-I/ARB 24 hours before coronary angiography does not appear to influence the incidence of contrast-induced nephropathy in stable patients with CKD stages 3–4 (Rosenstock *et al.*, 2008). Haemodialysis performed immediately after contrast administration has been ineffective at reducing the incidence of contrast-induced nephropathy. This is likely due to the fact that kidney injury occurs rapidly after administration of contrast and haemodialysis reduces the effective circulating volume and may itself be nephrotoxic by activation of inflammatory pathways.

Gupta R, Bang TJ. Prevention of contrast-induced nephropathy (CIN) in interventional radiology practice. Semin Intervent Radiol. 2010;27(4):348–59.

KDIGO. KDIGO Clinical Practice Guideline for acute kidney injury. Kidney Int Suppl. 2012;2:4.

Rosenstock JL, Bruno R, Kim JK, et al. The effect of withdrawal of ACE inhibitors or angiotensin receptor blockers prior to coronary angiography on the incidence of contrast-induced nephropathy. Int Urol Nephrol. 2008;40(3):749–55.

Weisbord SD, Gallagher M, Jneid H, et al.; PRESERVE Trial Group. Outcomes after angiography with sodium bicarbonate and acetylcysteine. N Engl J Med. 2018;378:603–14.

41. E. Thrombotic microangiopathy.

This patient most likely has developed cancer drug-induced thrombotic microangiopathy (TMA). Gemcitabine and mitomycin C are known to cause type 1 drug-induced TMA that is dose-related and with a delayed onset of 6–12 months after starting therapy. Unfortunately, there is a high probability of recurrence that precludes reintroduction at a later stage. There is also a high incidence of mortality (4-month mortality of up to 75%) and ESRD requiring dialysis despite drug discontinuation. This contrasts with anti-VEGF therapy that causes type 2 drug-induced TMA, with a much higher likelihood of recovery and better kidney survival rates after stopping the medication. ADAMTS-13 of >10% makes secondary aHUS/TMA likely.

Glezerman I, Kris MG, Miller V, et al. Gemcitabine nephrotoxicity and hemolytic uremic syndrome: report of 29 cases from a single institution. Clin Nephrol. 2009;71(2):130–9.

Izzedine H, Perazella MA. Thrombotic microangiopathy, cancer, and cancer drugs. Am J Kidney Dis. 2015;66(5):857–68.

42. C. Malignancy.

Malignancy accounts for around 35% of patients presenting to the emergency department with symptomatic hypercalcaemia. The commonest associated cancers include squamous cell cancers of the head/neck/lung, breast cancer, renal cell cancer, lymphoma, and myeloma. The types of cancer-associated hypercalcaemia include humoral hypercalcaemia of malignancy (due to overproduction of PTH-related peptide (PTHrP), 80%), release of local osteolytic factors (20%), and secretion of $1,25-(OH)_2$ vitamin D by the tumour (<1%). PTHrP shares the N-terminal end with PTH and can bind to the same receptor—type I PTH receptor. PTHrP can simulate most of the actions of PTH, including increased bone resorption, distal tubular calcium reabsorption, and inhibition of proximal tubular phosphate reabsorption. The clinical and laboratory findings are not consistent with the other options.

Lameire N, Van Biesen W, Vanholder R. Electrolyte disturbances and acute kidney injury in patients with cancer. Semin Nephrol. 2010 Nov;30(6):534–47.

Schlüter KD. PTH and PTHrP: Similar structures but different functions. News Physiol Sci. 1999 Dec;14:243–9.

43. E. Urinary alkalinization.

This patient fits the diagnostic criteria for tumour lysis syndrome (TLS). Risk factors for TLS include large tumour mass, potential for cell lysis, underlying CKD, volume depletion, and concurrent nephrotoxin exposure. Urinary alkalinization is no longer recommended for the management of TLS. Although urinary alkalinization increases the solubility of uric acid in the urine, it requires an adequate GFR with large urinary volumes to prevent acute urate nephropathy. This will not work in this scenario and could be potentially harmful. Increasing the urinary pH can enhance calcium phosphate crystal deposition, resulting in acute phosphate nephropathy and hypoxanthine/xanthine crystal deposition within the renal tubules. Rasburicase, intravenous hydration, and allopurinol are safe therapeutic options. Although allopurinol reduces further uric acid production, it will not correct hyperuricaemia. It could also increase the levels of hypoxanthine and xanthine levels, leading to their precipitation in renal tubules.

Cairo MS, Bishop M. Tumour lysis syndrome: new therapeutic strategies and classification. Br J Haematol. 2004 Oct;127(1):3–11.

Humphries BD, Sanders PW. Cancer and the kidney. ONF NephSAP. 2013;12(1). https://www.asn-onl ine.org/education/nephsap/volume.aspx?v=12

Richette P, Bardin T. Successful treatment with rasburicase of a tophaceous gout in a patient allergic to allopurinol. Nat Clin Pract Rheumatol. 2006 Jun;2(6):338–42; quiz 343.

44. C. Light chain deposition disease.

AKI, anaemia, hypercalcaemia with low PTH, and non-albumin proteinuria (trace protein on urine dipstick with an elevated protein:creatinine ratio) are important pointers to the diagnosis of an underlying plasma cell dyscrasia. Such a rapid decline in renal function is not in keeping with diabetic nephropathy or hypertensive nephrosclerosis. There are no clinical features consistent with pauci-immune glomerulonephritis. Adequate renal perfusion on Doppler ultrasound goes against a diagnosis of renal infarction. This patient would require a bone marrow biopsy, serum protein electrophoresis/immunofixation, 24-hour urine protein electrophoresis/immunofixation, and serum free light chains to confirm the diagnosis of multiple myeloma and to determine clonality to plan for clone-directed therapy. Biopsy would likely reveal nodular glomeruli with mesangial hypercellularity (PAS+ nodules) on light microscopy, kappa or lambda light chain positivity on immunofluorescence, and powdery/granular deposits in glomerular and tubular basement membranes on electron microscopy.

Korbet SM, Schwartz MM. Multiple myeloma. J Am Soc Nephrol. 2006;17(9):2533–45.

Wang Q, Jiang F, Xu G. The pathogenesis of renal injury and treatment in light chain deposition disease. J Transl Med. 2019 Nov 25;17(1):387. doi:10.1186/s12967-019-02147-4.

45. E. Thrombotic microangiopathy.

Vascular endothelial growth factor (VEGF) is produced by podocytes and VEGF receptors are present on the glomerular endothelium, mesangium, and peritubular capillaries. VEGF promotes angiogenesis and maintains vascular tone and fenestrated endothelium of the glomerular capillaries. Anti-VEGF therapy is used in malignancies, diabetic retinopathy, and age-related macular degeneration. Thrombotic microangiopathy is the commonest renal manifestation of anti-VEGF nephropathy. In a series of six patients treated with bevacizumab for various malignancies (Eremina et al., 2008), 100% developed thrombotic microangiopathy, 50% developed hypertension, and 50% had proteinuria. VEGF knockout mice (podocyte gene only) also demonstrated similar clinical, laboratory, and histological findings. Renal findings improved on withdrawal of bevacizumab. Onion skinning from hypertensive nephrosclerosis is unlikely to develop within 6 weeks.

Eremina V, Jefferson JA, Kowalewska J, *et al*. VEGF inhibition and renal thrombotic microangiopathy. N Engl J Med. 2008 Mar 13;358(11):1129–36.

Zhu X, Wu S, Dahut WL, Parikh CR. Risks of proteinuria and hypertension with bevacizumab, an antibody against vascular endothelial growth factor: systematic review and meta-analysis. Am J Kidney Dis. 2007 Feb;49(2):186–93.

46. A. Acute interstitial nephritis.

Immune checkpoint inhibitors are drugs that work by blocking checkpoint proteins, allowing T cells to attack and kill cancer cells. They are monoclonal antibodies that find and attach to a specific antigen on cancer cells. Tumour cells produce ligands such as PD-L1 and PD-L2, which bind to the PD-1 receptor (on the T-cell surface) and inactivate T cells. Pembrolizumab releases T cells from this inhibition, thereby exerting its anti-tumour effect. The commonest renal manifestation of immune checkpoint inhibitor-induced renal injury is acute interstitial nephritis, followed by acute tubular necrosis and minimal change disease. Treatment includes stopping the checkpoint inhibitor and other culprit medications and corticosteroids. Recurrence on re-exposure remains a possibility.

Cortazar FB, Marrone KA, Troxell ML, *et al*. Clinicopathological features of acute kidney injury associated with immune checkpoint inhibitors. Kidney Int. 2016 Sep;90(3):638–47.

Izzedine H, Escudier B, Lhomme C, *et al*. Kidney diseases associated with anti-vascular endothelial growth factor (VEGF): an 8-year observational study at a single center. Medicine (Baltimore). 2014 Nov;93(24):333–9. Erratum in: Medicine (Baltimore). 2014 Nov;93(24):414.

Shirali AC, Perazella MA, Gettinger S. Association of acute interstitial nephritis with programmed cell death 1 inhibitor therapy in lung cancer patients. Am J Kidney Dis. 2016 Aug;68(2):287–91.

47. D. Necrotizing glomerulonephritis with crescents.

Cocaine contaminated with levamisole (also known as levamisole-adulterated cocaine (LAC)) is associated with ANCA-associated vasculitis (both MPO and PR3). Levamisole is an anti-helminth that is used to cut cocaine and potentiates euphoria. Patients typically present with constitutional symptoms, cutaneous vasculitis with/without pulmonary haemorrhage, and pauci-immune focal necrotizing glomerulonephritis with crescents and ANCA positivity (usually MPO, but 50% can also be PR3-positive). Treatment includes cessation of the drug, BP control, and immune-modulating therapy for rapidly progressive glomerulonephritis. Hepatitis C-related membranoproliferative glomerulonephritis is unlikely in the context of sustained viral remission. There is no evidence of microangiopathic haemolytic anaemia or thrombocytopenia to suggest thrombotic microangiopathy. Minimal change disease and membranous nephropathy would be associated with nephrotic syndrome.

Pendergraft WF 3rd, Herlitz LC, Thornley-Brown D, Rosner M, Niles JL. Nephrotoxic effects of common and emerging drugs of abuse. Clin J Am Soc Nephrol. 2014 Nov 7;9(11):1996–2005.

48. B. Hydroxyethyl starch.

This patient most likely developed osmotic nephropathy and tubular injury from hydroxyethyl starch. Other causes of osmotic nephropathy include IVIg sucrose, volume expanders such as dextran 40, mannitol, and radiocontrast agents. Risk factors for osmotic nephropathy include underlying CKD, sepsis, and high doses of volume expanders. AKI results from reabsorption of hydroxyethyl starch via pinocytosis into the proximal tubular cells. This leads to hydropic swelling of the phagolysosome, followed by swelling and vacuolization of the proximal tubular epithelial cells. Vancomycin-induced nephrotoxicity is due to acute tubular necrosis and/or cast nephropathy. Ramipril causes haemodynamic pre-renal AKI; sepsis leads to acute tubular necrosis, and high-dose furosemide can result in acute interstitial nephritis. None of these, however, are associated with the morphological finding of osmotic nephropathy.

Brunkhorst FM, Engel C, Bloos F, et al. German Competence Network Sepsis (SepNet). Intensive insulin therapy and pentastarch resuscitation in severe sepsis. N Engl J Med. 2008 Jan 10;358(2):125–39.

Myburgh JA, Finfer S, Bellomo R, et al. CHEST Investigators; Australian and New Zealand Intensive Care Society Clinical Trials Group. Hydroxyethyl starch or saline for fluid resuscitation in intensive care. N Engl J Med. 2012 Nov 15;367(20):1901–11.

49. E. Urinary alkalinization.

Urinary alkalinization increases the excretion of salicylates by trapping the drug in the tubular lumen. This can be achieved by an intravenous bicarbonate infusion, with a target urinary pH of 7.5. Acidaemia increases central nervous system salicylate toxicity, and if ventilatory support is required, care must be provided to maintain high minute ventilation and elevated blood pH. According to The Extracorporeal Treatments In Poisoning Workgroup (EXTRIP) guidelines, extracorporeal treatment is recommended if any of the following are met:

- Salicylate level >7.2 mmol/L
- Salicylate level >6.5 mmol/L in the presence of impaired renal function
- Altered mental status
- New hypoxaemia requiring supplemental oxygen.

This patient does not meet any of the above criteria and thus does not qualify for renal replacement therapy. Intravenous fluid and furosemide will not achieve urinary alkalinization.

Juurlink DN, Gosselin S, Kielstein JT, et al. EXTRIP Workgroup. Extracorporeal Treatment for Salicylate Poisoning: Systematic Review and Recommendations From the EXTRIP Workgroup. Ann Emerg Med. 2015 Aug;66(2):165–81.

50. A. Aristolochic acid nephropathy.

Aristolochic acid nephropathy (also known as Chinese herb nephropathy) is caused by Chinese herbal slimming regimens (weight loss regimens) containing aristolochic acid (AA) where *Aristolochia fangchi* is substituted for *Stephania tetrandra*. Exposure to AA is also associated with urothelial malignancies. AA has been identified as the environmental agent causing Balkan-endemic nephropathy. The clinical presentation is consistent with progressive interstitial nephritis, bland urine sediment, and interstitial fibrosis and tubular atrophy. Biopsy findings (negative immunofluorescence and electron microscopy) and absence of proteinuria make diabetic nephropathy and focal segmental glomerulosclerosis unlikely. Histopathological findings are consistent with chronic changes.

Debelle FD, Vanherweghem JL, Nortier JL. Aristolochic acid nephropathy: a worldwide problem. Kidney Int. 2008 Jul;74(2):158–69.

Perazella MA, Luciano RL. Review of select causes of drug-induced AKI. Expert Rev Clin Pharmacol. 2015;8(4):367–71.

Take-Home Messages

1. CRRT modality: no one modality of CRRT is better than another (CVVHDF vs CVVHD vs CVVH) in terms of mortality benefit and overall survival. The choice of one over another would depend on patient characteristics, local expertise, available resources, and organizational aspects.

2. CRRT dose: there is no benefit to 'intensive' therapy. An effluent flow of at least 20–25 mL/kg/h is sufficient, with careful attention to ensuring that the target dose of therapy is actually delivered. To ensure delivery of the target dose, a prescription of 25–30 mL/kg/h may be needed.

3. CRRT anticoagulation: findings of citrate toxicity include worsening metabolic acidosis, increasing calcium infusion requirements, decreasing systemic ionized calcium, and a calcium ratio (total calcium/ionized calcium ratio) (also referred to as the calcium gap) of >2.5:1.

4. Intra-abdominal compartment syndrome should be considered as a diagnostic possibility in the context of AKI with blunt abdominal trauma and massive abdominal distension. Diagnosis can be made by measurement of intra-abdominal pressure with a urinary catheter.

5. As CRRT accelerates nutritional losses and contributes to protein malnutrition, daily protein intake should be increased to 1.5–2.5 g/kg/day to reach a positive nitrogen balance.

6. Systematic reviews and meta-analyses have shown an association between piperacillin–tazobactam and vancomycin combination therapy and an increased incidence of AKI.

7. The KDIGO Clinical Practice Guidelines recommend using volume expansion with either isotonic sodium chloride or sodium bicarbonate in patients at risk of contrast-induced AKI.

8. Thrombotic microangiopathy can be a manifestation of treatment with cancer chemotherapy. It is important to recognize the differences between type 1 and type 2 drug-induced thrombotic microangiopathy, as they portend varying prognoses and survival rates.

9. Malignancy-associated hypercalcaemia can be due to humoral hypercalcaemia of malignancy (PTHrP-related), release of local osteolytic factors, and secretion of $1,25\text{-(OH)}_2$ vitamin D.

10. Immune checkpoint inhibitors are an important and emerging cause for drug-induced AKI. The commonest renal manifestation of immune checkpoint inhibitor-induced renal injury is acute interstitial nephritis, followed by acute tubular necrosis, and minimal change disease.

11. Urinary alkalinization is no longer recommended for treatment of tumour lysis syndrome. Increasing urinary pH decreases uric acid precipitation but also enhances calcium phosphate crystal deposition (acute phosphate nephropathy) and hypoxanthine/xanthine crystal deposition within the renal tubules. It requires an adequate GFR with large urinary volumes to prevent/reduce acute urate nephropathy.

chapter 3

DISORDERS OF FLUID, ELECTROLYTES, AND ACID BASE

QUESTIONS

51. You are asked to see a 75-year-old woman admitted to hospital last night feeling generally unwell. She has a long history of mental health problems and is known to the psychiatry team; she had been treated with different anti-psychotics in the past. Nurses noticed that she was drinking a lot of water; however, they could not measure her urine output.

On examination, her BP was 120/75 mmHg and she was euvolaemic.

Investigations:

serum sodium	156 mmol/L (137–144)
serum potassium	4 mmol/L (3.5–4.9)
serum chloride	110 mmol/L (95–107)
serum creatinine	70 µmol/L (60–110)
random plasma glucose	5.6 mmol/L (3.0–11.1)
urine osmolality	200 mOsm/kg (100–1000)

What is the next best investigation for her hypernatraemia?

A. serum aldosterone
B. desmopressin test
C. morning urine cortisol
D. plasma osmolality
E. water deprivation test

Best of Five MCQs for the European Specialty Examination in Nephrology. Shafi Malik, Oxford University Press.
© Oxford University Press 2024. DOI: 10.1093/oso/9780192844163.003.0005

52. **An 85-year-old patient was brought to the emergency department from a nursing home due to altered mental status which started 2 days ago. She is diabetic, with good glycaemic control with use of metformin, and has no other significant past medical history. She was conscious but could not give the correct date, time, or place.**

    On examination, her pulse was 110 beats/min and her BP was 100/60 mmHg. There were no neurological deficits, and she had no oedema.

    Investigations:
serum sodium	156 mmol/L (137–144)
serum creatinine	145 µmol/L (60–110)
random plasma glucose	5.5 mmol/L (3.0–11.1)
serum urea	11 mmol/L (2.5–7.0)
urine osmolality	900 mOsm/kg (100–1000)

    What is the next best management step?

    A. rapid correction using 5% dextrose
    B. slow correction using 5% dextrose
    C. rapid correction using oral free water
    D. slow correction using oral free water
    E. rapid correction using 0.45% saline

53. **A 70-year-old man presented to the emergency department complaining of headache, nausea, and vomiting, which started a week ago. He has a past history of ischaemic heart disease, heart failure, and hypertension. He does not smoke or drink alcohol but says that he drinks a lot of tea. He was taking furosemide, nebivolol, pravastatin, aspirin, and ramipril.**

    On examination, he looked dehydrated and there was no lower limb oedema. His pulse was 110 beats/min and his BP was 100/50 mmHg.

    Investigations:
serum sodium	118 mmol/L (137–144)
serum urea	15 mmol/L (2.5–7.0)
serum creatinine	140 µmol/L (60–110)
random plasma glucose	5 mmol/L (3.0–11.1)
urine osmolality	300 mOsm/kg (100–1000)

    CT scan of the brain was normal.

    What is the best next step?

    A. 0.9% normal saline
    B. stop furosemide
    C. stop furosemide and give 3% hypertonic saline
    D. stop furosemide and give sodium chloride tablets
    E. 0.45% normal saline

54. **A 30-year-old lady was seen in the renal clinic with a history of muscle weakness. She had no significant past history and was not taking any regular medications, other than an occasional painkiller and a weight-losing pill.**

On examination, her weight was 50 kg, height 170 cm, pulse 100 beats/min and regular, and BP 100/60 mmHg. She was thin and had global muscular weakness, with no other neurological deficit.

Investigations:

serum urea	2.8 mmol/L (2.5–7.0)
serum sodium	140 mmol/L (137–144)
serum potassium	2.9 mmol/L (3.5–4.9)
serum bicarbonate	32 mmol/L (20–28)
random plasma glucose	5 mmol/L (3.0–11.1)
urine potassium	60 mmol/L (25–120)

Renin and aldosterone levels were significantly elevated.

What is the most probable cause of her hypokalaemia?

A. alkalosis

B. diuretic use

C. laxative abuse

D. low potassium diet

E. primary hyperaldosteronism

55. **A 60-year-old man was brought to the emergency department complaining of muscular weakness. He had a past history of heart failure, diabetes, and ESRD. He was taking enalapril, aspirin, pravastatin, and insulin.**

On examination, his pulse was 80 beats/min and his BP was 160/85 mmHg. He had lower limb oedema up to the knees bilaterally.

Investigations:

serum urea	20 mmol/L (2.5–7.0)
serum creatinine	540 µmol/L (60–110)
serum potassium	7.5 mmol/L (3.5–4.9)
serum sodium	135 mmol/L (137–144)
serum bicarbonate	18 mmol/L (20–28)

ECG showed narrow peaked T waves, with a prolonged PR interval.

What should be the most urgent management step?

A. 8.4% bicarbonate

B. calcium gluconate

C. haemodialysis

D. haemofiltration

E. patiromer

56. **A 40-year-old man was admitted to the psychiatric ward for acute psychosis. He is known to have mental health problems for many years and has been on long-term lithium treatment. He is also known to have hypertension and is taking ramipril and nebivolol.**

> **On examination, his BP was 130/80 mmHg and there was no peripheral oedema.**

> Investigations:
> serum creatinine   180 µmol/L (60–110)
> serum adjusted calcium   3.15 mmol/L (2.20–2.60)
> urine calcium   low
> plasma parathyroid hormone   18.7 pmol/L (0.9–5.4)
> serum protein   75 g/L (61–76)
> serum albumin   45 g/L (37–49)

What is the most likely cause of his hypercalcaemia?

A. dehydration
B. lithium
C. multiple myeloma
D. primary hyperparathyroidism
E. ramipril

57. **A 50-year-old man was brought to the emergency department by the police with altered sensorium. He was found on the street in an inebriated state. He is a known alcoholic, with no other significant past history.**

> **On examination, his GCS was 12, pulse 110 beats/min, and BP 110/60 mmHg. He had hyperreflexia, and Trousseau and Chvostek signs were positive.**

> Investigations:
> serum urea   2 mmol/L (2.5–7.0)
> serum albumin   27 g/L (37–49)
> serum adjusted calcium   1.75 mmol/L (2.20–2.60)
> serum magnesium   0.2 mmol/L (0.75–1.05)
> plasma parathyroid hormone   17.4 pmol/L (0.9–5.4)

What is the most probable cause of his hypocalcaemia?

A. alcohol
B. dehydration
C. hypomagnesaemia
D. malnutrition
E. vitamin C deficiency

58. **A 55-year-old man is seen in clinic for bone pain that started many weeks ago. He is a chronic haemodialysis patient, who was switched 6 months ago from thrice-weekly hemodialysis sessions to five times weekly long overnight hemodialysis in order to better control his hypertension and volume overload. He exercises regularly. However, he has not been able to do so lately due to bone pain.**

Investigations (before a dialysis session):
serum adjusted calcium   2.1 mmol/L (2.20–2.60)
serum phosphorus   0.5 mmol/L (0.80–1.45)
plasma parathyroid hormone   8.2 pmol/L (0.9–5.4)
serum 25-OH-cholecalciferol   99.8 nmol/L (50–120)

What is the most probable cause of his pains?

A. adynamic bone disease
B. hypophosphataemia
C. metastatic bone lesions
D. renal osteodystrophy
E. rheumatoid arthritis

59. **A 25-year-old man attended the renal clinic complaining of cramps and fatigue. His symptoms started many months ago with cramps in the arms and legs, which were sometimes severe, in addition to chronic fatigue. He also mentioned that he urinated a lot and got up twice at night to urinate.**

On examination, his BP was 105/60 mmHg and he was euvolaemic.

Investigations:
serum potassium   3 mmol/L (3.5–4.9)
serum chloride   95 mmol/L (95–107)
serum bicarbonate   35 mmol/L (20–28)
serum magnesium   0.3 mmol/L (0.75–1.05)
serum adjusted calcium   2.20 mmol/L (2.20–2.60)
urine calcium   low

What is the most likely diagnosis?

A. Bartter syndrome
B. Gitelman syndrome
C. hypocalcaemia due to hypomagnesaemia
D. malnutrition
E. surreptitious vomiting

60. **An 80-year-old man was seen in the emergency department with a history of diarrhoea and altered mental status. His past history included hypertension and Sjögren's syndrome. He was taking amlodipine and hydrochlorothiazide.**

    On examination, his pulse was 110 beats/min with a regular rhythm and his BP was 90/55 mmHg.

    Investigations:
serum creatinine	90 μmol/L (60–110)
serum sodium	138 mmol/L (137–144)
serum potassium	3.8 mmol/L (3.5–4.9)
serum bicarbonate	12 mmol/L (20–28)
serum chloride	118 mmol/L (95–107)
urine anion gap	low

    What is the most likely cause of his acidosis?

    A. acute kidney injury
    B. diarrhoea
    C. diuretics
    D. lactic acidosis
    E. renal tubular acidosis

61. **A 30-year-old man was brought to the emergency department for altered mental status. He is known to have insulin-dependent diabetes and is reported to be non-compliant with his treatment regimen. His brother, who brought him to the emergency department, said that the patient had been experiencing diarrhoea for past 2 days.**

    On examination, his GCS was 13, BP 100/60 mmHg, and respiratory rate 20 breaths/minute. He appeared dehydrated.

    Investigations:
serum sodium	140 mmol/L (137–144)
serum potassium	3.8 mmol/L (3.5–4.9)
serum chloride	110 mmol/L (95–107)
serum bicarbonate	8 mmol/L (20–28)
random plasma glucose	30 mmol/L (3.0–11.1)
blood ketones	positive

    What is the most likely cause for his acidosis?

    A. alcohol
    B. diabetes
    C. diabetes and diarrhoea
    D. diarrhoea
    E. starvation

62. **During a round on a haemodialysis unit, you were asked to review the case of a 50-year-old man who has been on haemodialysis for the past 2 years. His past history included ischaemic heart disease, hypertension, and diabetes, and he was taking calcium acetate, bisoprolol, aspirin, and insulin.**

    Investigations:
    serum adjusted calcium   2.5 mmol/L (2.20–2.60)
    serum phosphorus   2.5 mmol/L (0.80–1.45)
    plasma parathyroid hormone   26.5 pmol/L (0.9–5.4)
    serum bicarbonate   22 mmol/L (20–28)
    Kt/V   1.2

    What is the next most appropriate step?

    A. aluminium
    B. cinacalcet
    C. increase calcium acetate
    D. increase dialysis duration
    E. sevelamer

63. **A 40-year-old man was brought to the emergency department with confusion. He was conscious, but confused and drowsy. The patient is known to be an alcoholic, with no other medical problems.**

    On examination, his BP was 100/60 mmHg and his respiratory rate was 20 breaths/min. There was no neurological deficit.

    Investigations:
    serum urea   2 mmol/L (2.5–7.0)
    serum sodium   135 mmol/L (137–144)
    serum chloride   100 mmol/L (95–107)
    serum bicarbonate   15 mmol/L (20–28)
    random plasma glucose   7 mmol/L (3.0–11.1)
    plasma lactate   1 mmol/L (0.6–1.8)
    osmolality gap   normal

    What is the most likely cause of his acidosis?

    A. malnutrition
    B. diabetic ketoacidosis
    C. ethylene glycol intoxication
    D. lactic acidosis
    E. methanol intoxication

64. **A 60-year-old lady was admitted to the ICU following a tonic–clonic seizure. She was intubated and ventilated to protect her airways.**

    On examination, she appeared dehydrated. Her BP was 100/80 mmHg, and her temperature was 38.7°C.

    Investigations:
serum creatinine	300 μmol/L (60–110)
platelet count	30×10^9/L (150–400)
serum haptoglobin	low

    ADAMTS-13 was awaited. In the meantime, the patient was started on steroids and plasmapheresis with fresh frozen plasma.

    One week later, she was off ventilation and repeat tests showed:

platelet count	200×10^9/L (150–400)
serum haptoglobin	normal
serum bicarbonate	38 mmol/L (20–28)
pH	7.47 (7.35–7.45)†

    †(see Appendix II for pH/H+ conversion)

    ### What is the most likely cause of the alkalosis?

    A. haemolytic anaemia
    B. hypovolaemia
    C. mechanical ventilation
    D. plasmapheresis
    E. steroids

65. **A 70-year-old woman was referred to the renal clinic by her cardiologist for abnormal blood tests. Her past history included CKD stage 3, ischaemic heart disease, peptic ulcer, and hypertension. She was taking ramipril, calcium carbonate supplements, vitamin D, and furosemide. She reported no symptoms, except for abdominal pain and dyspepsia.**

    On examination, she was euvolaemic and her BP was 110/80 mmHg.

    Investigations:
serum adjusted calcium	3.1 mmol/L (2.20–2.60)
serum phosphate	0.9 mmol/L (0.80–1.45)
serum bicarbonate	37 mmol/L (20–28)
total protein	60 g/L (0.15–0.45)
plasma parathyroid hormone	low
serum 25-OH-cholecalciferol	125 nmol/L (50–120)

    ### What is the most likely explanation for the laboratory findings?

    A. multiple myeloma
    B. furosemide
    C. milk-alkali syndrome
    D. vitamin D intoxication
    E. vomiting

51. B. Desmopressin test.

This patient most likely has diabetes insipidus (DI), taking into account her apparent euvolaemia and low urine osmolality. If the ADH axis and renal response are intact, then urine osmolality should be above 600 mOsm/kg in the case of hypernatraemia. DI can be neurogenic or nephrogenic. Nephrogenic DI can be congenital or acquired. Acquired nephrogenic DI may be secondary to hypokalaemia, hypercalcaemia, and post-obstructive diuresis, as well as due to medications such as demeclocycline, lithium, foscarnet, or amphotericin. In this case, lithium-induced nephrogenic DI and neurogenic DI should be considered as a cause of her hypernatraemia. The water deprivation test would be useful to distinguish between DI and polydipsia in the case of polyuria. If the urine osmolality increases once the serum sodium level is above 145 mEq/L or serum osmolality is above 295 mOsm/L, then polydipsia is the diagnosis. Our patient has already a high serum sodium and low urine osmolality, so the water deprivation test will not be useful. Desmopressin will distinguish neurogenic from nephrogenic DI. If the urine osmolality increases in response to desmopressin administration, then neurogenic DI is the diagnosis. Hyperaldosteronism and Cushing's disease are not probable in this patient, as she has no hypertension or peripheral oedema. Causes of acquired central DI are post-trauma, post-surgery, tumours, histiocytosis, and granulomas such as sarcoidosis and tuberculosis.

Christ-Crain M, Winzeler B, Refardt J. Diagnosis and management of diabetes insipidus for the internist: an update. J Intern Med. 2021;290(1):73–87.

52. B. Slow correction using 5% dextrose.

This is chronic hypernatraemia with neurological symptoms and requires serum sodium correction slowly by 10 mmol/L, and not more than 12 mmol/L, over 24 hours. It can be achieved by administering 5% dextrose at 1.35 mL/kg/h, in addition to a volume equivalent to ongoing water losses if there are any. In general, a net positive balance of 3 mL of electrolyte-free water per kilogram of lean body weight will lower the serum sodium level by approximately 1 mmol/L. Serum sodium level should be checked every 6 hours in the first 24 hours. Oral free water administration could be used; however, it is not the best option in this patient with neurological symptoms. Acute hypernatraemia is treated more aggressively by giving IV 5% dextrose at a rate of 3–6 mL/kg/h, aiming to compensate for the whole water deficit in 24 hours. Serum sodium level should be monitored every 3 hours until it reaches 145 mEq/L, when the infusion rate is lowered to 1 mL/kg/h.

Using 0.45% saline solution to correct hypernatraemia is possible, although not in this case. It may be an option in the case of hypernatraemia due to hyperglycaemia and hypovolaemia in a patient with diabetic ketoacidosis or a hyperosmolar hyperglycaemic state. Hypernatraemia is expected in such cases because of an osmotic shift of water from extracellular fluid into cells. Using 0.45% saline is preferred due to ongoing urinary losses of sodium and water that are associated with glycosuria. Amiloride, thiazide diuretics, and a low-solute regimen can be useful in the case of nephrogenic DI.

Muhsin SA, Mount DB. Diagnosis and treatment of hypernatremia. Best Pract Res Clin Endocrinol Metab. 2016;30(2):189–203.

53. C. Stop furosemide and give 3% hypertonic saline.

This patient has symptomatic hyponatraemia, probably medication-related. One way to approach hyponatraemia is to classify it as hypotonic, isotonic, or hypertonic, according to serum osmolality. Hypertonic hyponatraemia may be seen in hyperglycaemia and IVIg or mannitol administration. Isotonic hyponatraemia may be seen in the case of high lipid or protein levels. In the case of hypotonic hyponatraemia, if the urine osmolality is <100 mOsm/kg, then the aetiology could be polydipsia, tea consumption, or beer potomania.

If the urine osmolality is >100 mOsm/L, then the volume status can be a clue to the cause. If euvolaemic, SIADH is the most probable cause. If hypovolaemic, then volume depletion is probably the cause. Heart failure, cirrhosis, or nephrotic syndrome may be the origin of hyponatraemia in the case of volume overload. Urine osmolality of above 100 mOsm/L makes heart failure and diuretic treatment potential causes. In this case, however, as the patient appears clinically dry, diuretic would be the most likely cause. Besides temporarily holding diuretics, 3% hypertonic saline should be used to manage this hyponatraemia because it is symptomatic. The goal of initial therapy is to raise the serum sodium concentration by 4–6 mmol/L in a 24-hour period. The maximum rate of correction should be 8 mmol/L in any 24-hour period to avoid osmotic demyelination syndrome.

Sterns RH, Hix JK, Silver SM. Management of hyponatremia in the ICU. Chest. 2013;144(2):672–9.

54. B. Diuretic use.

This patient has hypokalaemia due to diuretic use. Hypokalaemia could be the result of low potassium intake, potassium intracellular shift, or excess potassium losses. Low potassium intake would induce kidney reabsorption and a low urinary potassium level (<20 mmol/day). Intracellular potassium shift could be due to alkalosis, insulin, beta-adrenergic agents, thyrotoxicosis, hypothermia, or refeeding syndrome. Excess potassium losses might be through the GI tract or due to urinary losses. In GI losses, the urinary potassium level is normally low, as the kidney tries to reabsorb as much potassium as possible to achieve a normal serum potassium level, as in the case of laxative abuse. Gastric secretions contain a small amount of potassium. However, alkalosis due to gastric losses (vomiting or suction through a nasogastric tube), in addition to aldosterone secretion induced by the resulting hypovolaemia, would stimulate potassium secretion in the distal tubule, causing hypokalaemia. The kidney may lose potassium via different mechanisms. When the urinary potassium level is high, then aldosterone and renin levels should be measured.

Causes of hypokalaemia and elevated aldosterone levels are:

1. Hypertensive: renovascular disease and renin-secreting tumours
2. Hypo- or normotensive: diuretics, upper GI losses, or salt wasting nephropathies.

High urinary potassium levels with low aldosterone levels may be seen in Liddle syndrome.

In this patient, diuretic use is the most likely explanation, as the BMI and BP are low and the urinary potassium level is high. She also has alkalosis due to hypovolaemic hyperaldosteronism.

Unwin RJ, Luft FC, Shirley DG. Pathophysiology and management of hypokalemia: a clinical perspective. Nat Rev Nephrol. 2011;7(2):75–84.

55. B. Calcium gluconate.

Clinical manifestations of hyperkalaemia include muscle weakness and cardiac arrhythmias. If there are ECG changes, immediate treatment should include IV calcium gluconate to stabilize the cellular membrane potential as a cardioprotective measure against arrhythmias, in addition to shifting potassium into the intracellular space by using insulin with dextrose and beta-2 agonists. Correcting acidosis will have a limited effect in shifting potassium into the cellular space, but it may increase the renal excretion of potassium. Potassium binders can be used in addition.

Palmer BF, Clegg DJ. Diagnosis and treatment of hyperkalemia. Cleve Clin J Med. 2017;84(12):934–42.

56. B. Lithium.

This patient has lithium-induced hypercalcaemia. Long-term treatment with lithium can induce hypercalcaemia by lowering the sensitivity of calcium receptors in the parathyroid gland, which increases the calcium level required to suppress parathyroid hormone (PTH) secretion. In this case, there is hypercalcaemia, normal or mild PTH elevation, and low urinary calcium concentration. Hypercalcaemia might be the result of increased bone resorption, increased calcium absorption, or reduced calcium excretion. The approach to management of hypercalcaemia starts with measuring the PTH level. If it is high or abnormally normal, then we may suspect primary hyperparathyroidism, or low calcium receptor sensitivity such as medication-induced (lithium) or in familial hypocalciuric hypercalcaemia (where the urinary calcium level is low, in contrast to primary hyperparathyroidism). Primary hyperparathyroidism is not the most probable diagnosis in our patient, as usually the urinary calcium level is not low in primary hyperparathyroidism. Dehydration might cause hypercalcaemia by reducing renal calcium excretion, and we would expect the PTH level to be low.

Minisola S, Pepe J, Piemonte S, Cipriani C. The diagnosis and management of hypercalcaemia. BMJ. 2015;350:h2723.

57. C. Hypomagnesaemia.

Hypocalcaemia might be the result of hypomagnesaemia. Low magnesium level will create PTH resistance that would result in a hypocalcaemic state. Furthermore, severe hypomagnesaemia decreases PTH secretion from the parathyroid gland. In addition, magnesium therapy produces a rise in PTH secretion that occurs significantly earlier than restoration of PTH responsiveness. Alcohol can cause hypocalcaemia indirectly, due to pancreatitis or hypoalbuminaemia for example, or through hypomagnesaemia, in this patient, low magnesium may be related to malnutrition. Malnutrition can cause hypocalcaemia indirectly secondary to low magnesium and low albumin levels. However, it is not the direct cause in this case. Low calcium with low PTH can be due to genetic disorders affecting the parathyroid glands, surgical, autoimmune diseases, iron overload, radiation, or infections (HIV). Low Ca level with high PTH is the result of any cause of hypocalcaemia not directly affecting the parathyroid glands, which will create a PTH increase as a natural response.

Ayuk J, Gittoes NJ. Treatment of hypomagnesemia. Am J Kidney Dis. 2014;63(4):691–5.

58. B. Hypophosphataemia.

Hypophosphataemia may result from phosphorus redistribution into cells from the extracellular space, increased phosphate excretion, or reduced phosphate intestinal absorption. Hypophosphataemia can cause weakness, dysarthria, paraesthesia, confusion, seizures, osteomalacia, and coma. This patient has hypophosphataemia due to his intensive dialysis programme. Renal osteodystrophy can cause bone pains, but in this case, it is not the most likely cause as the PTH level is not very high and the symptoms started following modification to the dialysis regimen. The other options are unlikely.

Felsenfeld AJ, Levine BS. Approach to treatment of hypophosphatemia. Am J Kidney Dis. 2012;60(4):655–61.

59. B. Gitelman syndrome.

Bartter and Gitelman syndromes (also called tubular hypomagnesaemia–hypokalaemia with hypocalciuria) are autosomal recessive disorders with characteristic sets of metabolic abnormalities and are typical normotensive, salt-losing hypokalaemia tubulopathies. Electrolyte abnormalities include hypokalaemia, metabolic alkalosis, hyperreninaemia, hyperplasia of the juxtaglomerular apparatus, and hyperaldosteronism. The primary defect in both Bartter and Gitelman syndromes is impairment in one of the transporters involved in sodium chloride reabsorption in the loop of Henle or distal tubule. Hypomagnesaemia due to renal magnesium wasting can occur in both disorders but is a more prominent feature of Gitelman syndrome. Urinary calcium excretion is normal or high in patients with Bartter syndrome, as it is with a loop diuretic, since calcium reabsorption in the thick ascending limb requires normal sodium chloride reabsorption at this site. By contrast, urinary calcium excretion is typically reduced in patients with Gitelman syndrome, as it is with a thiazide diuretic. The most helpful laboratory test to distinguish vomiting from Gitelman syndrome is measurement of the urinary chloride concentration. This is usually <25 mEq/L in patients with chronic vomiting because of hypovolaemia and hypochloraemia. Hypocalcaemia due to hypomagnesaemia cannot explain the other electrolyte abnormalities in this patient.

Konrad M, Nijenhuis T, Ariceta G, et al. Diagnosis and management of Bartter syndrome: executive summary of the consensus and recommendations from the European Rare Kidney Disease Reference Network Working Group for Tubular Disorders. Kidney Int. 2021;99(2):324–35.

60. B. Diarrhoea.

This patient has a non-anion gap (AG) metabolic acidosis with a normal kidney response, as the urine AG is low. Serum $AG = Na - (Cl + HCO_3)$; it should be <12. If we add potassium to the equation, then the AG is increased by 4 (<16):

$$Serum\ AG = (Na + K) - (Cl + HCO_3)$$

Metabolic acidosis can be categorized as:

1. Non-AG: where there is loss of bicarbonate or impaired acid excretion.

   The two main causes are GI losses of bicarbonate and proximal or distal renal tubular acidosis. To see the difference, one can calculate the urine AG:

   $$Urine\ AG = (Na + K) - Cl$$

   It is normally slightly high, and it becomes low when the chloride concentration increases, as ammonium is eliminated in greater amounts in the urine to compensate for the acidosis (normal renal response).

2. AG acidosis: which might be the result of accumulation of either an intrinsic or an extrinsic acid substance.

   AKI can cause acidosis; however, it is not the most likely cause here. Sjögren's syndrome can cause renal tubular acidosis, but in that case, the urine AG would be more likely high. Lactic acidosis is a high AG acidosis.

Fenves AZ, Emmett M. Approach to patients with high anion gap metabolic acidosis: core curriculum 2021. Am J Kidney Dis: 2021;78(4):590–600.

61. C. Diabetes and diarrhoea.

This patient has two concomitant acidoses. One is diabetic ketoacidosis, which is a high AG acidosis. Serum $AG = Na - (Cl + HCO_3)$. In this case, the AG is 22. Ketones are positive and he is hyperglycaemic. However, this is not the only acidosis that he has, because the delta AG (delta AG is the excess AG, i.e. calculated AG minus expected AG) is less than the delta bicarbonate gap, which means that there is an additional reason that is causing a low bicarbonate level without having an impact on the AG, and in this case, it is the diarrhoea. Delta $AG = 22 - 12 = 10$. Delta HCO_3 = normal HCO_3 – patient's $HCO_3 = 23 - 8 = 15$. The delta AG would equal the delta bicarbonate gap in a pure high AG acidosis. If the delta AG is less than the delta bicarbonate gap, this means that there is an associated non-AG metabolic acidosis. If the delta AG is greater than the delta bicarbonate gap, then this means that there is an associated metabolic alkalosis. Starvation and alcohol can cause ketoacidosis.

Pandey DG, Sharma S. Biochemistry, anion gap. In: *StatPearls*. Treasure Island, FL: StatPearls Publishing; 2022. Available from: https://www.ncbi.nlm.nih.gov/books/NBK539757/

62. E. Sevelamer.

The best option for this patient is to switch to a non-calcium-based phosphate binder such as sevelamer or lanthanum. Vascular calcification in dialysis patients is a cardiovascular risk factor. This patient has a high normal serum calcium level with hyperphosphataemia and an elevated PTH level. Using a calcium-based phosphate binder will reduce the phosphataemia, but it might add a positive calcium load, which may increase the risk of vascular calcification. Increasing the dialysis session duration has a limited effect on phosphate level. However, increasing the haemodialysis session frequency would be useful. Cinacalcet will have a very limited effect in this case, as the PTH level is in the target level. Aluminium is rarely used due to the risk of neurological toxicity.

Scialla JJ, Kendrick J, Uribarri J, et al. State-of-the-art management of hyperphosphatemia in patients with CKD: an NKF-KDOQI controversies perspective. Am J Kidney Dis. 2021;77(1):132–41.

63. A. Malnutrition.

This patient has a high AG metabolic acidosis related to a poor nutritional state. Ethylene glycol and methanol intoxications would have presented with a high osmolality gap. Calculated serum osmolality $Sosm = (2 \times [serum\ Na\ in\ mmol/L]) + ([glucose\ in\ mg/dL]/18) + ([blood\ urea\ nitrogen\ in\ mg/dL]/2.8)$. Or, using SI units (mmol/L): calculated $Sosm = (2 \times [serum\ Na]) + [glucose] + [urea]$. An elevated serum osmolality gap exists if the measured osmolality is 10 mOsm/L greater than the calculated osmolality. High glucose levels are usually associated with diabetic ketoacidosis. Lactic acidosis is a high AG metabolic acidosis. However, the lactate level is normal in this case.

Brubaker RH, Vashisht R, Meseeha M. High anion gap metabolic acidosis. In: *StatPearls*. Treasure Island, FL: StatPearls Publishing; 2022. Available from: https://www.ncbi.nlm.nih.gov/books/NBK448090/

64. D. Plasmapheresis.

This patient has a metabolic alkalosis due to citrate in the FFP. Sodium citrate is metabolized to sodium bicarbonate, which is considered an alkali load. This alkali load is not excreted in patients with renal dysfunction. Steroids can rarely cause metabolic alkalosis through their mineralocorticoid effect; however, it is not the most likely cause here. Mechanical ventilation can cause a respiratory alkalosis if the parameters are adjusted to induce hyperventilation. Haemolytic anaemia would result in a metabolic acidosis.

Ijaz M, Abbas N, Lvovsky D. Severe uncompensated metabolic alkalosis due to plasma exchange in a patient with pulmonary-renal syndrome: a clinician's challenge. Case Rep Crit Care. 2015;2015:802186.

65. C. Milk-alkali syndrome.

The milk-alkali syndrome triad consists of hypercalcaemia, metabolic alkalosis, and renal insufficiency associated with ingestion of calcium and absorbable alkali. Calcium-induced diuresis results in volume depletion, which stimulates renal tubular absorption of bicarbonate. The combined effects of increased alkali intake, volume depletion, and decreased GFR lead to metabolic alkalosis. Volume depletion due to vomiting or diuretics will also worsen hypercalcaemia and alkalosis. Older patients have a reduced capacity for bone buffering, which may cause them to be at higher risk of hypercalcaemia following ingestion of calcium-containing supplements. Patients who appear to be at higher risk of milk-alkali syndrome include older individuals and those susceptible to volume depletion (including patients on thiazide diuretics). Hypophosphataemia is common, reflecting both the absence of a phosphate load, in conjunction with the calcium load, and the phosphate-binding properties of calcium carbonate. Historically, milk supplied the calcium load in milk-alkali syndrome. However, milk contains a large amount of phosphate, so hypophosphataemia would not develop in that case. Multiple myeloma can cause hypercalcaemia and acute kidney failure, but it is less likely here as the total protein level is normal. Vomiting can cause hypokalaemia, alkalosis, and hypercalcaemia due to hypovolaemia. However, it is not the most likely cause here. Vitamin D supplements can increase calcium but are associated with hyperphosphataemia.

Irtiza-Ali A, Waldek S, Lamerton E, Pennell A, Kalra PA. Milk alkali syndrome associated with excessive ingestion of Rennie: case reports. J Ren Care. 2008;34(2):64–7.

Take-Home Messages

1. Acquired nephrogenic DI may be secondary to hypokalaemia, hypercalcaemia, and post-obstructive diuresis, as well as due to medications such as demeclocycline, lithium, foscarnet, and amphotericin.
2. The desmopressin test will distinguish between neurogenic and nephrogenic DI.
3. Hypertonic hyponatraemia may be seen in hyperglycaemia and IVIG or mannitol administration. Isotonic hyponatraemia may be seen in the case of high lipid or protein levels.
4. Hypotonic hyponatraemia: if the urine osmolality is <100 mOsm/kg, then polydipsia, tea consumption, or beer potomania can be the cause. If the urine osmolality is >100 mOsm/kg and the patient is euvolaemic, SIADH is likely; if the patient is hypovolaemic, volume depletion is the likely cause; if there is volume overload, heart failure, cirrhosis, or nephrotic syndrome can be the origin.
5. To manage symptomatic hyponatraemia, 3% hypertonic saline should be used. The goal of initial therapy is to raise the serum sodium concentration by 4–6 mmol/L in a 24-hour period.
6. Bartter and Gitelman syndromes (also called tubular hypomagnesaemia–hypokalaemia with hypocalciuria) are autosomal recessive disorders and typical normotensive, salt-losing hypokalaemia tubulopathies. Electrolyte abnormalities include hypokalaemia and metabolic alkalosis.
7. Hypomagnesaemia is a prominent feature of Gitelman syndrome.
8. Serum $AG = (Na + K) - (Cl + HCO_3)$. Without potassium, it should be 12, and with potassium, it should be 16.
9. Lactic acidosis is a high AG acidosis.
10. Ethylene glycol and methanol intoxications present with a high osmolality gap.
11. Citrate in FFP can cause metabolic alkalosis.
12. Milk-alkali syndrome consists of hypercalcaemia, metabolic alkalosis, and AKI.

chapter

4

CHRONIC KIDNEY DISEASE, HAEMATURIA, AND PROTEINURIA

QUESTIONS

66. A 70-year-old man was referred for investigation of blood and protein in the urine. He is known to have hypertension and type 2 diabetes mellitus complicated by retinopathy, which was treated with laser photocoagulation a year ago. He was taking insulin, ramipril, amlodipine, atorvastatin, and doxazosin. He drank 16 units of alcohol per week and smoked 10 cigarettes a day.

On examination, his BP was 151/88 mmHg and there was oedema to his mid shins.

Urinalysis showed blood 3+, protein 1+ confirmed on repeat testing.

Investigations:

serum creatinine	230 µmol/L (60–110)
haemoglobin A_{1c}	92 mmol/mol (20–42)
urinary protein:creatinine ratio	192 mg/mmol (<30)
ultrasound scan of abdomen	left kidney 9 cm, right kidney 8 cm, non-obstructed

What is the next most appropriate investigation?

A. CT renal angiography
B. cystoscopy
C. kidney biopsy
D. radioisotope renogram
E. renal MRI

Best of Five MCQs for the European Specialty Examination in Nephrology. Shafi Malik, Oxford University Press.
 DOI: 10.1093/oso/9780192844163.003.0007

67. **A 45-year-old woman presented with persistent non-visible haematuria 3 weeks after treatment for a urinary tract infection. She had a hysterectomy 3 years ago for menorrhagia. She had no other past history and took no regular medications. She was adopted at birth and had no contact with her biological family.**

    On examination, her BP was 124/69 mmHg.

    Repeat urinalysis showed blood 3+.

    Investigations:
    serum creatinine   51 µmol/L (60–110)
    urinary protein:creatinine ratio   7 mg/mmol (<30)
    ultrasound scan of abdomen   normal-sized, non-obstructed kidneys

    What is the most appropriate next step?

    A. annual serum creatinine
    B. audiometry
    C. cystoscopy
    D. kidney biopsy
    E. slit-lamp examination

68. **A 41-year-old woman of Kenyan descent presented to the clinic with non-visible haematuria on two separate occasions 3 weeks apart. This was detected following routine testing for insurance purposes. There was no family history of kidney disease.**

On examination, her BP was 154/95 mmHg.

Urinalysis showed blood 2+. She underwent a renal biopsy.

Investigations:

serum creatinine	68 μmol/L (60–110)
urinary protein:creatinine ratio	28 mg/mmol (<30)
ultrasound scan of abdomen	normal-sized, non-obstructed kidneys
renal biopsy	see image

(a)   (b)

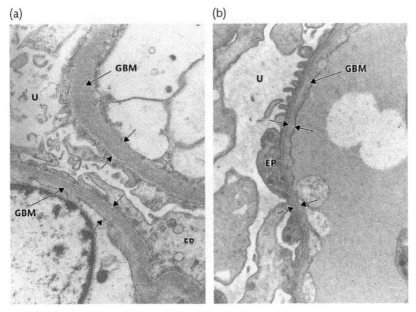

Reproduced with permission from Firth, John D., Peter Topham, and John Feehally (ed.), 'Thin membrane nephropathy', in John Firth, Christopher Conlon, and Timothy Cox (eds), *Oxford Textbook of Medicine*, 6 edn (Oxford, 2020; online edn, Oxford Academic, 1 Jan. 2020), https://doi.org/10.1093/med/9780198746690.003.0483.

What is the most appropriate first management step?

A. amlodipine

B. losartan

C. mycophenolate mofetil

D. prednisolone

E ramipril

69. **A 46-year-old man was found to have an abnormal urinalysis at an occupational medical examination. He was known to have hypertension treated with amlodipine.**

On examination, his BP was 143/78 mmHg.

Urinalysis showed blood 3+, protein 3+.

Investigations:

serum creatinine	143 µmol/L (60–110)
serum creatinine (6 weeks later)	148 µmol/L (60–110)
serum CRP	8 mg/L (<10)
urinary protein:creatinine ratio	292 mg/mmol (<30)
ultrasound scan of abdomen	normal-sized, non-obstructed kidneys
renal biopsy	see image

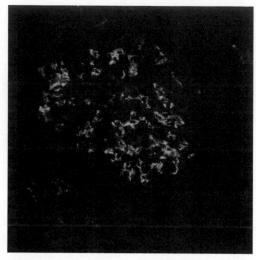

Immunofluorescence Reproduced with permission from Glassock, Richard J, Claudio Ponticelli, and Kar Neng Lai, 'Immunoglobulin A nephropathy', in Claudio Ponticelli, and Richard J. Glassock (eds), *Treatment of Primary Glomerulonephritis*, 3 edn, Oxford Clinical Nephrology Series (Oxford, 2019; online edn, Oxford Academic, 1 July 2019), https://doi.org/10.1093/med/9780198784081.003.0007.

What is the most appropriate first management step?

A. azathioprine

B. lisinopril

C. methylprednisolone

D. mycophenolate mofetil

E. rituximab

70. **A 48-year-old man with membranous nephropathy presented with a 1-week history of worsening peripheral oedema and weight gain. He had been treated with rituximab 18 months earlier and been in complete remission for the past 12 months. He had a serum creatinine level of 63 µmol/L 4 weeks prior to presentation.**

    On examination, his BP was 131/78 mmHg and there was oedema up to his mid thighs, with ascites and left-sided abdominal tenderness.
    Urinalysis showed blood 3+, protein 3+.

    Investigations:
serum creatinine	279 µmol/L (60–110)
serum albumin	21 g/L (37–49)
urinary protein:creatinine ratio	692 mg/mmol (<30)

    What is the most appropriate first treatment step?

    A. furosemide
    B. heparin
    C. lisinopril
    D. methylprednisolone
    E. rituximab

71. **A 22-year-old man was referred for investigation of proteinuria which had been identified at a routine employment medical check. He had a history of gastro-oesophageal reflux disease and was taking omeprazole.**

    On examination, he was euvolaemic and his BP was 121/73 mmHg.
    Urinalysis showed protein 2+.

    Investigations:
serum creatinine	61 µmol/L (60–110)
urinary protein:creatinine ratio	121 mg/mmol (<30)

    What is the next most appropriate investigation?

    A. albumin:creatinine ratio
    B. anti-PLA2R autoantibody
    C. first morning void protein:creatinine ratio
    D. renal biopsy
    E. serum IgA level

72. **A 65-year-old woman presented to hospital feeling generally unwell. She had been started on omeprazole, simvastatin, and aspirin 5 weeks previously following a TIA. Her serum creatinine level was 123 µmol/L and urinalysis was normal at the time.**

    On examination, her temperature was 37.1°C, BP 133/81 mmHg, respiratory rate 18 breaths/min, and oxygen saturations 97% on air. She had mild pedal oedema.

    Urinalysis showed protein 2+, leukocytes 1+.

    Investigations:
    serum creatinine   343 µmol/L (60–110)
    serum CRP   53 mg/L (<10)
    haemoglobin   115 g/dL (130–180)
    ultrasound scan of abdomen   normal-sized, non-obstructed kidneys

    ## What is the most likely mechanism of her proteinuria?

    A. functional proteinuria
    B. glomerular proteinuria
    C. orthostatic proteinuria
    D. overflow proteinuria
    E. tubular proteinuria

73. **A 76-year-old man presented with a 6-month history of progressive fatigue. He had type 2 diabetes mellitus, which was poorly controlled.**

On examination, his temperature was 37.6°C, BP 163/91 mmHg, respiratory rate 18 breaths/min, and oxygen saturations 97% on air. He was pale and had mild pedal oedema.

Urinalysis revealed blood 1+, protein 3+.

Investigations:
haemoglobin	72 g/L (115–165)
serum creatinine	443 µmol/L (60–110)
haemoglobin A_{1c}	92 mmol/mol (20–42)
urinary protein:creatinine ratio	632 mg/mmol (<30)
urinary albumin:creatinine ratio	120 mg/mmol (<2.5)
renal biopsy	see image

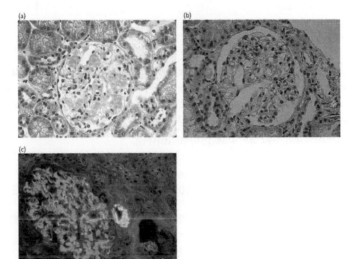

Reproduced with permission from Ronco, P, F Bridoux, and G Touchard, 'Renal involvement in plasma cell dyscrasias, immunoglobulin-based amyloidoses, and fibrillary glomerulopathies, lymphomas, and leukaemias', in David A. Warrell, Timothy M. Cox, and John D. Firth (eds), *Oxford Textbook of Medicine*, 5 edn, Oxford Textbooks (Oxford, 2010; online edn, Oxford Academic, 26 Nov. 2011).

What pathology is most likely to account for this presentation?

A. beta-2 microglobulin accumulation

B. elevated serum amyloid protein A

C. *JAK2* mutation

D. plasma cell dyscrasia

E. *V30M* mutation

74. **A 22-year-old man was found to have non-visible haematuria on a urine dipstick, performed during a routine medical assessment for enrolment in the armed forces. He had an active lifestyle and exercised every day. He denied any urinary tract symptoms, loin pain, fever, or episodes of visible haematuria. He had no past history or family history of kidney disease.**

    On examination, his BP was 124/76 mmHg.

    Investigations:
    serum creatinine   94 μmol/L (60–110)
    urinary protein:creatinine ratio   20 mg/mmol (<30)

    What is the most appropriate next step?

    A. abdominal ultrasound
    B. audiography
    C. autoantibody screen
    D. renal biopsy
    E. repeat urinalysis and urine microscopy

75. **A 26-year-old woman was referred with persistent non-visible haematuria. She was otherwise in good health. Her younger sister was evaluated several years earlier for the same problem, but no cause was found and she did not have a renal biopsy.**

    On examination, her BP was 110/60 mmHg.

    Investigations:
    serum creatinine   88 μmol/L (60–110)
    urinary protein:creatinine ratio   10 mg/mmol (<30)
    serum complement C3   109 mg/dL (65–190)
    urine microscopy   15–20 dysmorphic red cells
                                             no casts; <10 white blood cells

    What is the most likely cause of the haematuria?

    A. abnormal synthesis of $\alpha3/\alpha4$ chains of type IV collagen
    B. arteriovenous malformation of the renal artery
    C. *in situ* formation of immune complexes on the subepithelial side of the glomerular basement membrane
    D. mesangial deposition of immune complexes containing galactose-deficient IgA1
    E. mutation in the *LMX1B* gene

76. **A 37-year-old woman was referred for investigation of deteriorating renal function. She took ibuprofen occasionally for menstrual cramps and a herbal therapy for weight loss.**

    On examination, her BMI was 26 kg/m² and her BP was 134/82 mmHg.

    Investigations:

serum creatinine	289 µmol/L (60–110)
serum creatinine (6 months earlier)	87 µmol/L (60–110)
24-h urinary total protein	0.3 g (<0.2)
urine microscopy	8–10 red blood cells
	4–6 white blood cells
	no casts
ultrasound scan of abdomen	normal-sized kidneys with increased echogenicity

    ### What is a renal biopsy most likely to show?

    A. endocapillary hypercellularity

    B. focal segmental glomerulosclerosis

    C. interstitial inflammation and tubular atrophy

    D. interstitial non-caseating granulomas

    E. mesangial proliferation

77. **A 30-year-old woman presented with a short history of weight loss, low-grade fever, eye pain, and visual blurring.**

    On examination, her temperature was 37.8°C and her BP was 147/83 mmHg. There was bilateral redness of the eyes.

    Urinalysis revealed leukocytes 2+, protein 2+.

    Investigations:

serum creatinine	132 µmol/L (60–110)
urinary protein:creatinine ratio	30 mg/mmol (<30)
antinuclear antibody	1:160 (negative at 1:20 dilution)
serum complement C3	109 mg/dL (65–190)
haemoglobin	101 g/L (115–165)
MCV	86 fL (80–96)

    ### What is the most likely diagnosis?

    A. lupus nephritis

    B. microscopic polyangiitis

    C. mixed connective tissue disease

    D. sarcoidosis

    E. tubulointerstitial nephritis with uveitis syndrome

78. A 65-year-old woman with multiple myeloma was admitted for treatment of hypercalcaemia.

Investigations:

serum creatinine	110 µmol/L (60–110)
serum adjusted calcium	3.4 mmol/L (2.2–2.6)
urinary protein:creatinine ratio	50 mg/mmol (<30)

She was treated with intravenous 0.9% saline and intravenous pamidronate, and then commenced on regular pamidronate every 4–6 weeks.

At 12-month follow-up, investigations showed:

serum creatinine	256 µmol/L (60–110)
serum adjusted calcium	2.59 mmol/L (2.2–2.6)
urinary albumin:creatinine ratio	457 mg/mmol (<2.5)
urinary protein:creatinine ratio	610 mg/mmol (<30)

What is the most likely finding on renal biopsy?

A. acute interstitial nephritis
B. cast nephropathy
C. focal segmental glomerulosclerosis
D. membranous nephropathy
E. nodular glomerulosclerosis

79. A 22-year-old man from South Asia was referred with dysuria and an elevated creatinine level. He had recently moved to the UK with his family, having spent most of his life in Sri Lanka working as a farm labourer. He was taking no regular medications, and there was no family history of note.

His BP in clinic was 128/84 mmHg.

Urinalysis revealed protein 1+, leukocytes 2+.

Investigations:

serum creatinine	394 µmol/L (60–110)
serum creatinine (6 weeks ago)	385 µmol/L (60–110)
urinary protein:creatinine ratio	85 mg/mmol (<30)
ultrasound scan of abdomen	small kidneys bilaterally (<10 cm). No evidence of hydronephrosis

What further feature is most likely to suggest a diagnosis of CKD of unknown aetiology?

A. elevated creatinine kinase
B. hypermagnesaemia
C. hyperphosphataemia
D. hypoalbuminaemia
E. hypokalaemia

80. **A 38-year-old man was referred for evaluation of impaired renal function. He had suffered from gout for the past 10 years. His maternal grandfather had died of kidney failure and his mother started dialysis when she was 56 years old.**

Examination was unremarkable. His BP was 143/82 mmHg.
Urinalysis showed blood trace, protein 2+.

Investigations:
serum potassium	2.7 mmol/L (3.5–4.9)
serum creatinine	140 µmol/L (60–110)
serum urate	0.60 mmol/L (0.23–0.46)
urinary protein:creatinine ratio	46 mg/mmol (<30)
ultrasound scan of abdomen	normal-sized kidneys, single 2-cm cyst in the right kidney
MRI of abdomen	multiple small cysts, ranging from 3 mm to 2 cm, at the corticomedullary junction

What is the most likely diagnosis?

A. autosomal dominant polycystic kidney disease
B. autosomal recessive polycystic kidney disease
C. medullary cystic kidney disease
D. nephronophthisis
E. tuberous sclerosis

81. **A 41-year-old man was found to have non-visible haematuria at a routine health check. He had no past history of note and no family history of kidney disease.**

Examination was unremarkable and his BP was 156/91 mmHg.
Urinalysis revealed blood 2+.

Investigations:
serum creatinine	140 µmol/L (60–110)
urinary protein:creatinine ratio	6 mg/mmol (<30)

What would be the likely finding on a renal biopsy?

A. glomerular basement membrane thickening
B. glomerulomegaly
C. mesangial cell interposition
D. mesangial hypercellularity
E. podocyte hypertrophy

82. **A 71-year-old woman presented with shortness of breath, pleuritic chest pain, and oedema to her mid thighs. She was known to have type 2 diabetes mellitus and hypertension, and was taking metformin and amlodipine. A CT pulmonary angiogram showed a pulmonary embolus and she was started on therapeutic anticoagulation.**

    Investigations:
serum albumin	21 g/L (37–49)
serum creatinine	132 μmol/L (60–110)
urinary protein:creatinine ratio	1410 mg/mmol (<30)
haemoglobin	85 g/dL (100–120)

    What is the next most appropriate investigation?

    A. anti-cardiolipin antibodies
    B. anti-phospholipase A2 receptor antibody
    C. CT scan of the abdomen and pelvis
    D. renal biopsy
    E. serum free light chains

83. **A 59-year-old woman with CKD stage 3b, presumed to be due to diabetic nephropathy, attended the nephrology outpatient clinic for a routine review. Her past history included type 2 diabetes mellitus, essential hypertension, osteoarthritis, and dyslipidaemia. She was taking ramipril, amlodipine, atorvastatin, and insulin.**

    During the clinic appointment, she asked whether she required any specific vaccinations in view of her CKD.

    Which of the following vaccinations should she be advised to have?

    A. *Haemophilus influenzae* B
    B. hepatitis B
    C. herpes zoster
    D. yellow fever
    E. *Neisseria meningitidis*

84. **A 61-year-old woman with CKD stage 5 was due to have a colonoscopy following a positive faecal occult blood test. She continued to pass 2 L of urine a day. Her weight had been stable at 65 kg, with no change in her appetite.**

    On examination, her BP was 138/95 mmHg and there was no peripheral oedema.

    What is the most appropriate bowel cleansing preparation?

    A. bisacodyl
    B. magnesium citrate
    C. polyethylene glycol
    D. sodium phosphate
    E. sodium picosulfate

85. **A 71-year-old woman with CKD required a CT scan with contrast to investigate for possible malignancy. She had polymyalgia rheumatica and ischaemic heart disease.**

    On examination, there was oedema up to her mid shins.

    Investigations:
    eGFR   35 mL/min/1.73 m² (>60)
    echocardiogram   left ventricular ejection fraction 35%

    Which of the following is most appropriate to reduce the risk of contrast-induced nephropathy?

    A. intravenous 0.9% sodium chloride
    B. intravenous 1.26% sodium bicarbonate
    C. intravenous furosemide
    D. intravenous low-osmolar contrast medium
    E. intravenous N-acetylcysteine

86. **A 47-year-old man was found to have impaired renal function following investigation for non-specific low back pain.**

    On examination, his BP was 163/91 mmHg. Abdominal examination was unremarkable and there was bilateral pitting ankle oedema.

    Urine dipstick showed protein 2+, blood 1+, leukocytes 1+.

    Investigations:
    haemoglobin   112 g/L (130–180)
    white cell count   12.3 × 10⁹/L (4.0–11.0)
    serum creatinine   443 µmol/L (60–110)
    serum CRP   73 mg/L (<10)
    serum alkaline phosphatase   55 U/L (45–105)
    ultrasound scan of abdomen   bilateral hydronephrosis

    What feature makes retroperitoneal fibrosis the most likely diagnosis?

    A. abnormal urinalysis
    B. age at presentation
    C. elevated CRP
    D. normal abdominal examination
    E. normal alkaline phosphatase

87. **A 29-year-old woman presented with general malaise and breathlessness.**

    On examination, her BP was 169/97 mmHg and her oxygen saturations were 97% on room air. Her chest was clear on auscultation, and there was bilateral ankle oedema.

    Urine dipstick showed protein 2+, blood 3+.

    Investigations:
haemoglobin	110 g/L (115–165)
serum creatinine	943 µmol/L (60–110)
serum CRP	73 mg/L (<10)
ultrasound scan of abdomen	normal-sized, non-obstructed kidneys

    What associated finding is most likely to support a diagnosis of anti-GBM disease?

    A. eosinophilia
    B. hypocomplementaemia
    C. red cell casts on urine microscopy
    D. retinal haemorrhages
    E. vasculitic rash

88. **A 35-year-old man with CKD stage 4 due to vesicoureteric reflux attended the nephrology clinic. He asked about the likelihood of his children inheriting the condition. He had two brothers and two sisters; both of his brothers also had a history of vesicoureteric reflux.**

    How likely are his children to inherit vesicoureteric reflux?

    A. 25% of his children will be affected
    B. 50% of his children will be affected
    C. all boys will be affected
    D. all girls will be carriers
    E. there is an increased (but not quantifiable) risk of his children being affected

89. **A 42-year-old man with CKD stage 3 due to IgA nephropathy attended clinic for review. He smoked 30 cigarettes per day and was overweight, with a BMI of 40 kg/m^2. He was taking no regular medications.**

    On examination, his BP was 146/87 mmHg.

    Investigations:
    serum creatinine   150 μmol/L (60–110)
    serum cholesterol   5.8 mmol/L (<5.2)
    urinary protein:creatinine ratio   49 mg/mmol (<30)

    What is most likely to slow the progression of his CKD?

    A. cease smoking
    B. control BP to <130/80 mmHg
    C. reduce cholesterol concentration to <4 mmol/L
    D. reduce dietary sodium intake to <100 mmol/day
    E. weight reduction to a BMI of 20–25 kg/m^2

90. **A 27-year-old man presented with a 6-month history of polyuria and polydipsia, and 3 weeks of worsening shortness of breath on exertion. He had also experienced pain in both feet.**

    On examination, his BP was 164/84 mmHg. There were bibasal crepitations on auscultation of the chest, and he had a number of abdominal telangiectasias.

    Investigations:
    serum creatinine   270 μmol/l (60–110)
    urinary protein:creatinine ratio   320 mg/mmol (<30)

    A renal biopsy was performed.

    Which of the following is most likely to be found on electron microscopy?

    A. mesangial electron-dense deposits
    B. multilamellar myelin bodies in podocytes
    C. subepithelial electron-dense deposits
    D. tubular reticular inclusion bodies
    E. widespread foot process effacement

91. **An 18-year-old man was referred for investigation of persistent non-visible haematuria. His paternal uncle also had haematuria and deafness, and no one else in the family were affected.**

> **On examination, his BP was 122/66 mmHg. Physical examination was otherwise unremarkable.**
>
> Urinalysis showed blood 2+.
>
> Investigations:
> serum creatinine   61 μmol/L (60–110)
> urinary protein:creatinine ratio   7 mg/mmol (<30)
>
> Renal biopsy: 'Glomeruli appear normal on light microscopy. The glomerular basement membrane uniformly measures <200 nM on electron microscopy. Immunofluorescence reveals negative staining for IgG and C3, and there is positive staining for α3 and α5 collagen chains in the glomerular basement membrane and tubular basement membrane.'

What is the most likely diagnosis?

A. autosomal recessive Alport syndrome
B. branchio-oto-renal syndrome
C. nail patella syndrome
D. thin basement membrane nephropathy
E. X-linked Alport syndrome

92. **A 28-year-old man was referred for investigation of hypertension and impaired renal function. He had a 15-year history of well-controlled epilepsy and was taking sodium valproate and levetiracetam.**

> **Examination revealed hypopigmented areas of skin on the arms and trunk, and his BP was 156/104 mmHg.**
>
> Investigations:
> serum creatinine   151 μmol/L (60–110)
> urinary protein:creatinine ratio   7 mg/mmol (<30)
> ultrasound scan of abdomen   hyperechoic kidneys with several small cysts

Which form of surveillance should be commenced?

A. echocardiography
B. MRI scan of brain
C. ultrasound scan of kidneys
D. urinary acetyl phenylcitrate
E. urinary catecholamines

93. **A 35-year-old man presented with a 6-month history of intermittent abdominal pain. He had a 5-year history of gout. His maternal aunt had been on dialysis for 15 years before dying from a myocardial infarction. His mother had died in a road traffic accident when he was 3 years old. No other members of his family were known to have kidney disease.**

    On examination, his BP was 158/94 mmHg.

    Investigations:
serum creatinine	171 μmol/L (60–110)
ultrasound scan of abdomen	bilateral medullary cysts

    Which one of the following is most likely to be found?

    A. defective uromodulin secretion by the loop of Henle
    B. Tamm–Horsfall protein casts on urine microscopy
    C. increased fractional urate excretion
    D. low spot urinary sodium
    E. mutation in the *PKD2* gene

94. **A 19-year-old man was referred for evaluation of renal function impairment identified during a recent admission for investigation of palpitations.**

    Examination demonstrated clusters of small, dark red papules over the lower abdomen and thighs, which had become more extensive over the past 2 years. His BP was 145/85 mmHg.

    Investigations:
serum creatinine	131 μmol/L (60–110)
urinary protein:creatinine ratio	137 mg/mmol (<30)
ultrasound scan of abdomen	normal-sized kidneys; no obstruction

    Which investigation is most likely to confirm the diagnosis?

    A. glucagon test
    B. peripheral leukocyte cystine level
    C. plasma α-galactosidase A level
    D. serum galactose-1-phosphate level
    E. serum caeruloplasmin level

95. **A 25-year-old man presented with visible haematuria and ureteric colic. CT KUB demonstrated a stone in the distal right ureter. The stone passed spontaneously, with complete resolution of symptoms. He experienced a similar episode 9 months ago.**

    Investigations:

serum adjusted calcium	2.2 mmol/L (2.2–2.6)
serum phosphate	1.0 mmol/L (0.8–1.4)
24-h urinary calcium	3.0 mmol (2.5–7.5)
24-h urinary urate	2.0 mmol (<3.6)
24-h urinary oxalate	0.20 mmol (0.14–0.46)
24-h urinary cystine	550 μmol (<100)

    Which treatment is most likely to prevent further stone formation?

    A. acetazolamide

    B. allopurinol

    C. furosemide

    D. indapamide

    E. penicillamine

66. B. Cystoscopy.

This patient has established diabetes mellitus with microvascular complications. It is likely that he has diabetic nephropathy, accounting for CKD and proteinuria. Clinical findings that point towards a diagnosis other than, or in addition to, diabetic nephropathy include:

- absence of microvascular complications of diabetes mellitus
- nephrotic syndrome
- a sudden and significant rise in proteinuria or creatinine level
- persistent haematuria
- absence of proteinuria.

This patient has evidence of persistent non-visible haematuria, which could be suggestive of an inflammatory glomerular disorder. However, his age and smoking history raise the concern of a urological malignancy and should therefore be excluded.

Gonzalez Suarez ML, Thomas DB, Barisoni L, Fornoni A. Diabetic nephropathy: is it time yet for routine kidney biopsy? World J Diabetes. 2013;4(6):245–55.

National Institute for Health and Care Excellence (2021). Clinical Knowledge Summaries. Urological cancers – recognition and referral: symptoms suggestive of urological cancers. Available from: https://cks.nice.org.uk/topics/urological-cancers-recognition-referral/diagnosis/symptoms-suggestive-of-urological-cancers/

67. A. Annual serum creatinine.

This patient has persistent non-visible haematuria. The commonest differentials for this are:

- IgA nephropathy
- Alport disease
- thin basement membrane nephropathy.

Her underlying disease is at greater risk of progression to end-stage renal disease if any of the following are present:

- hypertension
- proteinuria
- impaired renal function.

Given she has none of these risk factors, her risk of progressive disease is low and further treatment is not required. A biopsy will not alter clinical management, regardless of the diagnosis. There are instances in which biopsies are indicated in such circumstances, including for employment purposes (e.g. in the armed forces) and during workup for kidney donation (where IgA nephropathy or severe Alport disease would be a contraindication, thin basement membrane nephropathy would not be a contraindication, however).

Despite her risk of progression being minimal, there is nevertheless a risk. It is therefore recommended that such patients have annual creatinine, BP, and urine dipstick checks under primary care, with advice to refer back to nephrology should any risk factors develop.

Hall CL, Bradley R, Kerr A, Attoti R, Peat D. Clinical value of renal biopsy in patients with asymptomatic microscopic hematuria with and without low-grade proteinuria. Clin Nephrol. 2004;62(4):267–72.

Vivante A, Afek A, Frenkel-Nir Y, et al. Persistent asymptomatic isolated microscopic hematuria in Israeli adolescents and young adults and risk for end-stage renal disease. JAMA. 2011;306(7):729–36.

68. A. Amlodipine.

This patient has persistent non-visible haematuria, with hypertension as a risk factor for progressive disease. Biopsy shows uniform thinning of the glomerular basement membrane (GBM) on electron microscopy (<250 nm). Differentials for this presentation are Alport disease and thin basement membrane nephropathy (TBMN). Both are disorders of the GBM.

Features suggestive of TBMN over Alport disease include:

- no family history of kidney disease
- no clinical features of Alport disease (proteinuria, hearing loss, retinopathy, and lenticonus)
- no *COL4A5* mutation (if genetic testing is performed)
- absence of a 'lamellated' appearance of the GBM
- normal α3 and α5 type IV collagen units on immunofluorescence.

This patient likely has TBMN. Management includes proteinuria control with ACE inhibitors or ARBs, and BP control. This patient has no evidence of proteinuria, so BP control would be key. Given her ethnicity, a calcium channel blocker would be the first line antihypertensive.

National Institute for Health and Care Excellence (2019, updated 2022). Hypertension in adults, diagnosis and management. NICE guideline [NG136]. Available from: https://www.nice.org.uk/guidance/ng136

Savige J, Gregory M, Gross O, Kashtan C, Ding J, Flinter F. Expert guidelines for the management of Alport syndrome and thin basement membrane nephropathy. J Am Soc Nephrol. 2013;24(3):364–75.

Tryggvason K, Patrakka J. Thin basement membrane nephropathy. J Am Soc Nephrol. 2006;17(3):813–22.

69. B. Lisinopril.

This patient has IgA nephropathy (IgAN), evidenced by mesangial IgA deposition, without IgM or C1q deposits. The renal biopsy contains fibrocellular crescents.

Risk factors for progressive IgAN are:

- proteinuria
- hypertension
- impaired renal function
- presence of any one of five histological findings described by the MEST-C score (also referred to as the Oxford Classification).

Components of the MEST-C score include:

- **M**esangial hypercellularity
- **E**ndocapillary hypercellularity

- **S**egmental glomerulosclerosis
- **T**ubular atrophy/fibrosis
- **C**rescents.

The risk of ESRD or creatinine level doubling in 5 years can be predicted by the IgAN prediction tool. IgAN management centres around renin-angiotensin system inhibition, BP control, and lifestyle optimization (dietary salt reduction, weight optimization, and smoking cessation). TESTING and STOP-IgAN trials found no benefit to immunosuppression in IgAN, but demonstrated side effects. Rituximab also has not been found to be beneficial in a randomized controlled trial. Immunosuppression can be used for IgAN presenting as rapidly progressive disease, defined as a decline in eGFR by >50% within 3 months. The presence of crescents warrants closer monitoring and vigilance for rapidly progressive disease, but should not on its own guide treatment.

Kidney Disease: Improving Global Outcomes (KDIGO) (2020). Chapter 2: Immunoglobulin A nephropathy/immunoglobulin A vasculitis. In: *KDIGO Clinical Practice Guideline on Glomerular Diseases*. Public review draft; pp. 109–32.

Selvaskandan H, Cheung CK, Muto M, Barratt J. New strategies and perspectives on managing IgA nephropathy. Clin Exp Nephrol. 2019;23(5):577–88.

70. B. Heparin.

This patient with membranous nephropathy has nephrotic syndrome and is at risk of venothromboembolic events (VTEs). VTEs in nephrotic syndrome can be driven by loss of antithrombotic factors in the urine and an increase in prothrombotic factors produced by the liver. VTEs associate mostly with nephrotic syndrome secondary to membranous nephropathy.

Features in keeping with a renal vein thrombosis (RVT) include:

- abdominal pain
- AKI
- blood and protein on urine dipstick.

RVTs can occur in up to 60% of patients with membranous nephropathy. AKI and active urinary sediment are thought to be driven by a sharp increase in intra-glomerular pressure.

Suspected RVTs should be treated with therapeutic anticoagulation, and the diagnosis confirmed by CT and MRI of the renal vessels. Screening for VTEs in nephrotic syndrome is not currently recommended, but those who are hypoalbuminaemic should be started on therapeutic anticoagulation, directed by the underlying disease process and serum albumin levels.

Lin R, McDonald G, Jolly T, Batten A, Chacko B. A systematic review of prophylactic anticoagulation in nephrotic syndrome. Kidney Int Rep. 2019;5(4):435–47.

71. C. First morning void protein:creatinine ratio.

This young patient presents with isolated sub-nephrotic range proteinuria, with normal renal function and BP. The likelihood of significant or active disease is low. The most frequent cause of this presentation among young adults and children is orthostatic proteinuria. It rarely presents above the age of 30. Orthostatic proteinuria resolves in the recumbent position such as in sleep. A first morning void urine sample which yields no evidence of proteinuria confirms the diagnosis. Even relatively brief periods of non-recumbence can induce orthostatic proteinuria, and thus counselling patients with regard to sample collection is critical for diagnosis.

The mechanisms governing orthostatic proteinuria are not clear. Postulations include increased intra-glomerular pressures secondary to entrapment of the left renal vein by the superior mesenteric artery and aorta ('nutcracker syndrome'), and heightened angiotensin II responses on standing. Follow-up of those with orthostatic proteinuria over four decades has demonstrated no risk of progressive kidney disease conferred by the diagnosis. It may resolve with age.

Nishizaki N, Obinata K, Nakagawa M, Shimizu T. Orthostatic proteinuria due to smartphone use in bed. Nephrology (Carlton). 2018;23(8):797.

Uehara K, Tominaga N, Shibagaki Y. Adult orthostatic proteinuria. Clin Kidney J. 2014;7(3):327–8.

72. E. Tubular proteinuria.

There is evidence of AKI, with no clear pre-renal causes and no evidence of obstructive uropathy. Her urine dipstick shows moderate proteinuria and leukocyturia, in the context of having recently started a proton pump inhibitor. This is in keeping with tubulointerstitial nephritis (TIN). TIN is an immune-mediated nephritis triggered by drugs (most commonly), infections, or autoimmune disorders. Triggers may generate an immune response through 'molecular mimicry' or by altering antigens found in the interstitium ('planted antigens'). The proteinuria that accompanies TIN is tubular, generated by tubular cell damage. It rarely exceeds 1.5 g/day.

TIN presents on a spectrum.

Symptoms may include:

- rash
- arthralgia
- loin pain.

Serum abnormalities may include:

- AKI
- eosinophilia
- thrombocytopenia
- anti-drug antibodies.

Urine abnormalities may include:

- proteinuria
- haematuria
- leukocyturia (eosinophiluria).

The only definitive way to diagnose TIN is by renal biopsy, which will demonstrate tubular–interstitial inflammation. TIN often resolves with removal of the offending drug or treatment of the underlying cause. Corticosteroids (often at 1 mg/kg/day) can be initiated, should renal function fail to recover despite this or renal replacement therapy-dependent AKI develops.

Joyce E, Glasner P, Ranganathan S, Swiatecka-Urban A. Tubulointerstitial nephritis: diagnosis, treatment, and monitoring. Pediatr Nephrol. 2017;32(4):577–87.

73. D. Plasma cell dyscrasia.

Biopsy shows amorphous material in the mesangium and capillary loops. On light microscopy, these may be mistaken for nodular glomerulosclerosis, pathognomonic of diabetic nephropathy. However, after staining with Congo red, apple green birefringence is demonstrated under polarized light, characteristic of amyloidosis.

Amyloidosis is an accumulation of proteins which misfold into fibrils. It can be secondary to various aetiologies, including myeloma, chronic inflammatory diseases, genetic mutations, and long-term haemodialysis.

Features in keeping with myeloma here are:

- renal function impairment
- anaemia
- evidence of overflow proteinuria (urine PCR much greater than urine ACR).

Other features of myeloma include hypercalcaemia and bone involvement. Diagnosis can be confirmed by testing for a paraprotein.

Myeloma is the driver of amyloidosis here, making plasma cell dyscrasia the explanation for the patient's presentation. Serum amyloid protein A accumulates secondary to chronic inflammatory diseases; beta-2 microglobulin is removed by the kidneys and thus accumulates in those receiving long-term haemodialysis without high-flux filters. *V30M* mutation is the commonest cause of hereditary amyloidosis. *JAK2* mutations are associated with polycythaemia rubra vera.

Dember LM. Amyloidosis-associated kidney disease. J Am Soc Nephrol. 2006;17(12):3458–71.

74. E. Repeat urinalysis and urine microscopy.

This patient has presented with a single episode of isolated non-visible haematuria. The most important next step is to establish if this is transient or persistent by repeat testing. Persistent non-visible haematuria of glomerular origin is commonly due to IgA nephropathy, Alport disease, or TBMN. Other causes may be urological (malignancy, infections, anatomical abnormalities, malformations) or systemic (hypertension, sickle cell and drug-induced papillary necrosis, clotting disorders). Transient haematuria can be driven by urinary tract infections, nephrolithiasis, or trauma or may be exercise-induced. Exercise-induced haematuria is a benign condition that requires no further management and is the most likely diagnosis in this case—if the haematuria is transient. The mechanism by which it occurs is not clear, but postulations include mild trauma to the bladder during exercise and an increase in capillary permeability mediated by lactic acid accumulation during exercise.

Jones GR, Newhouse I. Sport-related hematuria: a review. Clin J Sport Med. 1997;7(2):119–25.

75. A. Abnormal synthesis of $\alpha 3/\alpha 4$ chains of type IV collagen.

The commonest causes of non-visible haematuria are:

- IgA nephropathy
- Alport disease
- thin basement membrane nephropathy (TBMN).

Alport disease and TBMN are both disorders of the glomerular basement membrane (GBM), characterized by a uniformly thin GBM which occurs due to inherited abnormalities of the *COL4* genes for type IV collagen. Alport disease is more severe and is associated with:

- family history of kidney disease
- extra-renal manifestations (hearing loss, lenticonus)
- lamellation of the GBM on electron microscopy
- mutations of *COL4A5*.

Mutations involving *COL4A3* or *COL4A4* can be found in both Alport disease and TBMN. This is the most likely explanation for this presentation, given the family history. Although IgA nephropathy is a possibility (characterized by mesangial deposition of immune complexes containing galactose-deficient IgA), it is rarely inherited.

Savige J, Gregory M, Gross O, et al. Expert guidelines for the management of Alport syndrome and thin basement membrane nephropathy. J Am Soc Nephrol. 2013;24(3):364–75.

Yeo SC, Cheung CK, Barratt J. New insights into the pathogenesis of IgA nephropathy. Pediatr Nephrol. 2018;33(5):763–77.

76. C. Interstitial inflammation and tubular atrophy.

The patient's use of herbal therapy hints at a diagnosis of aristolochic acid nephropathy (AAN), supported by the subacute rise in creatinine level, with mild (likely tubular) proteinuria, leukocyturia, and non-visible haematuria. Aristolochic acid (AA) is a constituent of some herbal weight loss remedies. Its association with renal disease was first reported in a study from Belgium, and so it is also referred to as 'Balkan endemic nephropathy'. AAN typically causes hypocellular interstitial nephritis, with tubular atrophy and fibrosis being predominant features. Renal function recovery is therefore not always possible.

Ibuprofen causes acute interstitial nephritis; tubular atrophy is unlikely, unless exposure was sustained and prolonged. Non-caseating granulomas are commonly attributed to sarcoidosis and are only rarely associated with NSAID use. Focal segmental glomerulosclerosis is a podocytopathy and unlikely to present with non-visible haematuria or leukocyturia; the level of proteinuria would also be higher. Endocapillary hypercellularity and mesangial proliferation are findings often associated with lupus nephritis and IgA nephropathy. There are no clinical features suggestive of lupus, and the level of proteinuria will likely be higher if these lesions were present.

Debelle FD, Vanherweghem JL, Nortier JL. Aristolochic acid nephropathy: a worldwide problem. Kidney Int. 2008;74(2):158–69.

77. E. Tubulointerstitial nephritis with uveitis syndrome.

Tubulointerstitial nephritis with uveitis syndrome (TINU) is a form of acute interstitial nephritis (AIN) that presents with ophthalmological symptoms consistent with uveitis. It is an immune-mediated reaction presumed to be against an antigen common to the uvea and kidney. The mechanism by which it develops is unclear, but it appears to affect young women most frequently. TINU is diagnosed following a renal biopsy consistent with AIN and confirmation of a diagnosis of uveitis, which may require slit-lamp examination. TINU is largely self-limiting, and cases that do not resolve can be managed with corticosteroids.

The lack of haematuria makes lupus nephritis and microscopic polyangiitis unlikely, and C3 is often low in active lupus nephritis. There are also no overt clinical features to suggest lupus nephritis, microscopic polyangiitis, mixed connective tissue disease, or sarcoidosis.

Regusci A, Lava SAG, Milani GP, Bianchetti MG, Simonetti GD, Vanoni F. Tubulointerstitial nephritis and uveitis syndrome: a systematic review. Nephrol Dial Transplant. 2022;37(5):876–86.

78. C. Focal segmental glomerulosclerosis.

Pamidronate is a cause of drug-induced focal segmental glomerulosclerosis (FSGS), making this the most likely explanation for the development of proteinuria in this patient.

Acute interstitial nephritis (AIN) is unlikely, given the level of proteinuria. AIN results in tubular proteinuria that rarely exceeds 1.5 g/day. Cast nephropathy is unlikely, given the relatively similar levels of protein and albumin in the urine, suggesting the proteinuria is due to a glomerular leak instead of an overflow of immunoglobulins. Nodular glomerulosclerosis, also known as Kimmelstiel–Wilson lesions, are pathognomonic features of diabetic nephropathy, which is unlikely in this case, given there is no history of diabetes mellitus or associated microvascular complications. This leaves membranous nephropathy and FSGS as the remaining options, and given the history of exposure to pamidronate, FSGS is more likely than *de novo* membranous nephropathy.

Other drugs that can lead to secondary FSGS include opioids, anabolic steroids, calcineurin inhibitors, lithium, interferons, and sirolimus.

Resolution is possible with cessation of offending medications.

Rosenberg AZ, Kopp JB. Focal segmental glomerulosclerosis. Clin J Am Soc Nephrol. 2017;12(3):502–17. Erratum in: Clin J Am Soc Nephrol. 2018;13(12):1889.

Tucker BM, Luciano RL. Medication-associated glomerular disease. In: H Trachtman, L Herlitz, E Lerma, J Hogan, eds. *Glomerulonephritis*. Cham: Springer, 2019; pp. 735–72.

79. E. Hypokalaemia.

CKDu was first described in a cohort of Central American patients and is also known as mesoamerican nephropathy. Those affected are commonly young men who spend prolonged time working in agriculture and exposed to high temperatures.

Presentations include advanced kidney disease, muscle weakness and fatigue (caused by hypokalaemia), and sterile dysuria (caused by uric acid crystalluria). Electrolyte abnormalities characteristic of tubular dysfunction are present and include hypokalaemia, hyponatraemia, hypomagnesaemia, and hypophosphataemia. Hyperuricaemia is often present. Imaging reveals small kidneys bilaterally. Biopsies for this reason are rarely done, but those who present earlier have interstitial fibrosis and glomerular sclerosis with no immune deposits.

Diagnosis is made on the basis of a characteristic presentation and the absence of findings suggestive of another diagnosis (such as hyperglycaemia, hypertension, haematuria, nephrotic range proteinuria, cystic kidneys, and suggestive immunology).

The mechanisms governing the condition are not clear; recurrent heat stress is thought to contribute. The incidence of CKDu is increasing worldwide, with endemics reported in Africa and South Asia.

Treatment is limited to generic interventions for CKD, revolving around cardiovascular risk factor modification.

Campese VM. The unresolved epidemic of chronic kidney disease of uncertain origin (CKDu) around the world: a review and new insights. Clin Nephrol. 2021;95(2):65–80.

80. C. Medullary cystic kidney disease.

The MRI findings, history of gout, and autosomal dominant pattern of inherited kidney disease are suggestive of medullary cystic kidney disease (MCKD) due to a *UMOD* mutation.

MCKD, also known as autosomal dominant tubulointerstitial disease, develops due to mutations in:

- *UMOD* (commonest, codes for uromodulin and is associated with gout)
- *MUC1* (codes for mucin-1)
- *REN* (least common, codes for renin).

Uromodulin is synthesized at the loop of Henle where it maintains Na-K-2Cl activity. Failure disrupts sodium and water reabsorption, increasing reabsorption at the proximal tubules, which is accompanied by increased urate absorption. Kidney failure is related to tubular cell death due to uromodulin accumulation. MCKD can be diagnosed through a suggestive family history and genetic testing. Treatment is limited to generic interventions for CKD and gout.

The cysts of polycystic kidney are large and easily visualized by ultrasonography and involve both the cortex and the medulla of the kidney. Tuberous sclerosis is accompanied by extra-renal features. Nephronophthisis follows an autosomal recessive inheritance pattern and usually leads to ESRD by the second decade of life.

Bleyer AJ, Kidd K, Živná M, Kmoch S. Autosomal dominant tubulointerstitial kidney disease. Adv Chronic Kidney Dis. 2017;24(2):86–93.

81. D. Mesangial hypercellularity.

Impaired renal function and hypertension in the presence of non-visible haematuria increases the risk of progressive kidney disease; a biopsy and further management are warranted.

The commonest glomerular causes for this presentation are:

- IgA nephropathy (IgAN)
- Alport disease
- thin basement membrane nephropathy.

IgAN is the commonest of these and is diagnosed by dominant mesangial IgA ± IgG deposits, which may be accompanied by the presence of C3; mesangial hypercellularity is seen, making this the most likely finding on light microscopy. C1q and IgM will not be present, differentiating it from lupus nephritis. The remaining options are all associated with conditions that present with proteinuria.

Thickening of the glomerular basement membrane is seen in diabetic nephropathy, although it can also be feature of advanced membranous nephropathy. Glomerulomegaly is hypertrophy of the glomerulus which occurs in response to increased loads exerted on nephrons. It is usually secondary to systemic disorders such as obesity, structural heart disease, and congenital kidney malformations. It often accompanies focal segmental glomerulosclerosis.

Mesangial cell interposition is a prelude to 'double contouring', which refers to duplication of the glomerular basement membrane in response to immune complex deposits. It is seen in mesangioproliferative glomerulonephritis, lupus nephritis, and transplant glomerulopathy.

Podocyte hypertrophy is associated with diabetic nephropathy.

National Kidney Foundation. *AJKD Atlas of Renal Pathology.* Elsevier, 1999.

82. B. Anti-phospholipase A2 receptor antibody.

This patient has presented with a venothromboembolic event (VTE) in the context of nephrotic syndrome. Hypercoagulability occurs in nephrotic syndrome due to loss of anticoagulant proteins in the urine (antithrombin III and plasminogen) and an increase in prothrombotic proteins (I, VII, VIII, and X). VTEs in the context of nephrotic syndrome most often occur when membranous nephropathy (MN) is the underlying disease. Anti-phospholipase A2 receptor (PLA2R) antibodies are highly specific for primary MN (sensitivity 0.78, specificity 0.99) and account for 80% of cases. Seropositivity for this alone is sufficient for diagnosis in typical cases, allowing the risks associated with renal biopsy to be avoided. Anti-PLA2R is also a prognostic biomarker. Levels correlate with disease activity and can be used to monitor for treatment response, and those with elevated titres should be monitored closely for relapse.

Anti-thrombospondin type-1 domain-containing 7A (anti-THSD7A) antibodies are seen in 5% of primary MN cases, but this is yet to be validated as a diagnostic or prognostic tool in place of a renal biopsy.

The remaining cases of primary MN are likely mediated by antibodies that are currently being validated or are yet to be described.

Alsharhan L, Beck LH Jr. Membranous nephropathy: core curriculum 2021. Am J Kidney Dis. 2021;77(3):440–53.

Dahan K, Gillion V, Johanet C, Debiec H, Ronco P. The role of PLA2R antibody in treatment of membranous nephropathy. Kidney Int Rep. 2017;3(2):498–501.

83. B. Hepatitis B.

KDIGO guidelines recommend all adults with CKD at high risk of progressive disease be immunized against hepatitis B, with response confirmed by serological testing. Immunization is required due to the prevalence of hepatitis B among the haemodialysis population and the theoretical risk of transmission. Seroconversion rates are variable, diminishing with declining renal function. Determining those at risk of progressive CKD involves an evaluation of:

- the sustained change of eGFR from baseline
- the degree of albuminuria
- clinical factors (age, underlying diagnosis, sex, ethnicity, presence of hypertension, cardiovascular risk factors, lifestyle, and ongoing use of nephrotoxic agents).

If seroconversion has not been achieved (antibody levels <100 mIU), primary vaccination with three doses can be repeated. Antibody levels are monitored annually in those who receive haemodialysis. KDIGO guidelines also recommend those with CKD be offered annual influenza and pneumococcal vaccinations (for GFR categories G4–5 and those at high risk of pneumococcal infection, for example, those with nephrotic syndrome or diabetes, or receiving immunosuppression) every 5 years. *H. influenzae* B, herpes zoster, and *N. meningitidis* vaccines are not routinely recommended in CKD.

Kidney Disease: Improving Global Outcomes (KDIGO) CKD Work Group. KDIGO 2012 clinical practice guideline for the evaluation and management of chronic kidney disease. Kidney Int Suppl. 2013;3(1):1–50.

84. C. Polyethylene glycol.

Polyethylene glycol (PEG) is the recommended bowel preparation for CKD patients, provided they continue to pass good volumes of urine. PEG requires dissolution in large volumes of water (2–4 L), making it unsuitable for those at risk of fluid overload. The risk of electrolyte disturbances is lower, compared to other preparations. As this patient continues to pass good volumes of urine, a 2-L PEG regimen would be suitable. Magnesium salt preparations are relatively contraindicated in patients with CKD stages 4 and 5, and sodium picosulfate preparations should be used with caution. Both are associated with a risk of magnesium accumulation. Their use is reserved for those unable to tolerate the large volumes of fluid required with PEG. Sodium phosphate is not recommended for bowel preparation in CKD due to the potential risk of severe AKI (presumably due to acute phosphate nephropathy). CKD stages 3–5 is an absolute contraindication to sodium phosphate administration. Bisacodyl is not recommended as a bowel cleansing preparation.

Connor A, Tolan D, Hughes S, Carr N, Tomson C. Consensus guidelines for the safe prescription and administration of oral bowel-cleansing agents. Gut. 2012;61(11):1525–32.

Hassan C, East J, Radaelli F, et al. Bowel preparation for colonoscopy: European Society of Gastrointestinal Endoscopy (ESGE) guideline—update 2019. Endoscopy. 2019;51(8):775–94.

85. D. Intravenous low-osmolar contrast medium.

Low-osmolar contrast media and iso-osmolar contrast media are less nephrotoxic and recommended for those with pre-existing impairment of renal function. Current evidence suggests oral fluids are as good as intravenous fluids at preventing contrast-induced AKI, and there is no particular type of oral or intravenous fluids that is most effective. Only inpatients at particularly high risk of AKI need intravenous fluids. Risk factors include:

- CKD with eGFR <40 mL/min/1.73 m^2
- diabetes and eGFR <40 mL/min/1.73 m^2
- heart failure
- renal transplant
- age >75

- hypovolaemia
- high volume of contrast required
- arterial contrast with first-pass renal exposure.

Even though this patient has many of these risk factors, she is volume-overloaded. Fluid administration would not be appropriate in her case. Furosemide and mannitol are not correct, as forced euvolaemic diuresis leads to a significantly increased risk of contrast-induced nephropathy. The role of N-acetylcysteine (either oral or intravenous) to prevent contrast-induced nephropathy is not established. NICE AKI guidelines acknowledge the limited and mixed evidence base for this intervention, and neither recommend nor restrict its use for prevention of contrast-induced nephropathy.

Faggioni M, Mehran R. Preventing contrast-induced renal failure: a guide. Interv Cardiol. 2016;11(2):98–104.

National Institute for Health and Care Excellence (2019). Acute kidney injury: prevention, detection and management (evidence review for preventing contrast-induced acute kidney injury). NICE guideline [NG148]. https://www.nice.org.uk/guidance/ng148/chapter/Recommendations

86. C. Elevated CRP.

Retroperitoneal fibrosis can occur at any age, including childhood, but is most frequently reported between the ages of 40 and 60. It is also more common in men than in women (2:1). It is usually idiopathic and its pathophysiology has not been fully established. It is suspected to involve immune-mediated inflammation and fibrosis. It is associated with:

- HLA-B27
- other autoimmune diseases
- IgG4 disease.

Due to the ongoing inflammatory process, patients may experience systemic symptoms such as anorexia, fever, and weight loss. The encapsulating impact of a highly fibrotic retroperitoneum varies, and clinical features may include:

- pain (e.g. abdominal, back, flank, scrotal)
- oedema
- varicoceles and hydroceles
- obstructive uropathy and progressive kidney disease
- intestinal ischaemia, necrosis, and haemorrhage
- abdominal masses
- ascites.

Inflammatory markers, such as CRP and ESR, are typically raised in retroperitoneal fibrosis. Urinalysis is usually normal, as renal failure is due to an obstructive uropathy. There are case reports describing elevated alkaline phosphatase levels in association with retroperitoneal fibrosis. However, the nature of this association has not been established.

Vaglio A, Maritati F. Idiopathic retroperitoneal fibrosis. J Am Soc Nephrol. 2016;27(7):1880–9.

87. C. Red cell casts on urine microscopy.

Autoantibodies in anti-GBM disease target a hidden epitope within the $\alpha 3$ subunit of type IV collagen. This is most highly expressed in the:

- glomerular basement membrane
- alveolar basement membrane.

It has also been described in other tissues, including the:

- retina
- choroid plexus
- cochlea.

Anti-GBM disease usually presents as a rapidly progressive glomerulonephritis, and almost two-thirds of patients have concurrent alveolar haemorrhage. A minority will have isolated pulmonary disease. Disease involving other organs is inconsistently reported.

Involvement of the glomerular basement membrane leads to significant glomerular inflammation, resulting in extensive inflammatory cell infiltration. This gives rise to the histopathological finding of a crescent, which is an accumulation of inflammatory cells within Bowman's space. Glomerular inflammation leads to glomerular haematuria, which can be detected as non-visible haematuria on dipstick testing and as dysmorphic red blood cells on urine microscopy.

The other options are not commonly associated with anti-GBM disease. Although retinal haemorrhages have been rarely described concurrently with a presentation of anti-GBM disease, it is debated if this is driven by hypertensive retinal changes and/or anti-GBM antibodies. Management is with corticosteroids, cyclophosphamide, and plasma exchange, with the aim of rescuing patients from alveolar haemorrhage and ESRD. It is therefore not recommended for those who are dialysis-dependent on presentation, have an adequate biopsy demonstrating crescents in 100% of glomeruli (low probability of recovery), and have no pulmonary involvement. For those who are dialysis-dependent, it is recommended that transplantation be delayed by 6 months after antibody titres are undetectable, to minimize the risk of transplant recurrence.

McAdoo SP, Pusey CD. Anti-glomerular basement membrane disease. Clin J Am Soc Nephrol. 2017;12(7):1162–72.

88. E. There is an increased (but not quantifiable) risk of his children being affected.

Vesicoureteric reflux refers to the abnormal retrograde flow of urine from the bladder into the ureters and kidneys. This can result in recurrent episodes of acute pyelonephritis and subsequent reflux nephropathy, which can progress to ESRD. There is a clear genetic component highlighted by familial clustering of cases. However, genetic patterns are heterogenous and no single gene locus or gene has been identified. There is therefore an increased (but not quantifiable) risk of this patient being affected.

Diagnosis can be made through a voiding cystourethrogram. Treatment options include:

- prophylactic antibiotics
- open ureteric reimplantation
- endoscopic injection of dextranomer and hyaluronidase at the vesicoureteric junction
- laparoscopic ureteric reimplantation.

Nino F, Ilari M, Noviello C, et al. Genetics of vesicoureteral reflux. Curr Genomics. 2016;17(1):70–9.

89. B. Control BP to <130/80mmHg.

All the listed options are beneficial for a patient with IgA nephropathy. However, the evidence base is strongest for BP control. At the time of writing, there are no disease-specific treatments approved for treatment of IgA nephropathy. This is likely to change in the very near future. Currently, the only safe interventions proven to reduce the risk of progressive disease are:

1. maximal renin–angiotensin system (RAS) inhibition
2. BP control

3. salt reduction
4. weight optimization
5. smoking cessation
6. cardiovascular risk factor control.

The evidence base is strongest for RAS inhibition and BP control, which appear to confer prognostic benefits independent of each other.

Selvaskandan H, Cheung CK, Muto M, Barratt J. New strategies and perspectives on managing IgA nephropathy. Clin Exp Nephrol. 2019;23(5):577–88.

90. B. Multilamellar myelin bodies in podocytes.

The clinical history is suggestive of Fabry disease. Fabry disease is an X-linked lysosomal disorder due to a gene defect encoding the α-galactosidase A enzyme. This results in the accumulation of glycosphingolipids in the lysosomes of all tissues, including the kidney, contributing to the multisystem presentation.

Multilamellar myelin bodies in podocytes (also known as zebra bodies) are pathognomonic of Fabry disease and can be seen on electron microscopy. Zebra bodies are intralysosomal inclusion bodies that indicate the accumulation of phospholipids.

There are two phenotypes. The features of classic Fabry (type 1) disease are:

- childhood or adolescence presentation
- neuropathic pain
- anhidrosis or hypohidrosis
- gastrointestinal symptoms (abdominal pain, cramping, and frequent bowel movements)
- dermatological abnormalities (angiokeratomas and telangiectasia, characteristic corneal dystrophy that does not affect vision).

Classic Fabry disease will lead to CKD (which contributes to hypertension), cardiac abnormalities (arrhythmia, hypertrophy), and an increased risk of a cerebrovascular event.

In late-onset Fabry (type 2) disease, the patient presents with renal and cardiac abnormalities between 30 and 70 years old, with minimal other symptoms, due to residual enzyme activity.

Rizk D, Chapman AB. Cystic and inherited kidney diseases. Am J Kidney Dis. 2003;42(6):1305–17.

91. D. Thin basement membrane nephropathy.

Thin basement membrane nephropathy and Alport syndrome are inherited disorders of type IV collagen which leads to a uniformly thin glomerular basement membrane. Given this patient has no extra-renal manifestations, thin basement membrane nephropathy is the most likely diagnosis. Alport syndrome is most frequently X-linked (85% of cases) due to a defect in the gene encoding the α5 chain of type IV collagen (*COL4A5*). There are also autosomal dominant and autosomal recessive forms which can involve the *COL4A3*, *COL4A4*, or *COL4A5* genes. In contrast to thin basement membrane nephropathy, there are extra-renal manifestations (sensorineural deafness, ocular defects, leiomyomatosis of the oesophagus and genitalia) and a high risk of progressive renal function loss. Abnormalities on renal biopsy include lamellation of the lamina densa on electron microscopy and absence of α3, α4, or α5 chains on staining.

The clinical features are not in keeping with brachio-oto-renal syndrome and nail patella syndrome.

Rizk D, Chapman AB. Cystic and inherited kidney diseases. Am J Kidney Dis. 2003;42(6):1305–17.

92. B. MRI scan of brain.

The clinical history is suggestive of tuberous sclerosis complex. This is an autosomal dominant condition due to a defect in a tumour suppressor gene (*TSC1* or *TSC2*) resulting in multisystem involvement, including:

- renal (angiomyolipomas, cysts)
- skin (facial angiofibromas, ungual or periungual fibromas, shagreen patches, and hypomelanotic macules)
- ocular (retinal hamartomas)
- central nervous system (epilepsy, giant cell astrocytomas)
- cardiac (rhabdomyomas)
- pulmonary (multifocal micronodular pneumocyte hyperplasia).

MRI of brain every 1–3 years is recommended to identify and monitor sub-ependymal giant cell astrocytomas, or monitor those with a confirmed diagnosis of sub-ependymal giant cell astrocytoma without symptoms of raised intracranial pressure. MRI should be done more frequently for patients with a large or growing sub-ependymal giant cell astrocytoma, or those with a sub-ependymal giant cell astrocytoma causing ventricular enlargement but who remain asymptomatic. Ultrasound scan of kidney is not the preferred surveillance option. MRI of abdomen is recommended to assess for angiomyolipoma, renal cysts, or other renal lesions.

Surveillance with echocardiography is only recommended if the patient is known to have rhabdomyomas.

Tuberous Sclerosis Association (2019). UK guidelines for managing tuberous sclerosis complex. A summary for clinicians in the NHS. https://tuberous-sclerosis.org/for-professionals/healthcare-profes sionals/uk-clinical-guidelines-for-tsc/

93. A. Defective uromodulin secretion by the loop of Henle.

The clinical features of renal impairment, medullary cysts, and gout, together with the family history, are suggestive of medullary cystic kidney disease, an autosomal dominant disorder.

This is most commonly caused by mutations in the *UMOD* gene. As a result, the defective uromodulin proteins, which are restricted to the thick ascending limb of the loop of Henle, cannot exit the endoplasmic reticulum, resulting in cell death and progressive renal damage. In addition, defective uromodulin can lead to increased urate absorption and hyperuricaemia.

Medullary cystic kidney disease also occurs due to mutations in the *MUC1* (mucin-1) and *REN* (renin) genes.

A spot urinary sodium is not specific to a condition and is typically used in the evaluation of hyponatraemia. A mutation in the *PKD2* gene is responsible for autosomal dominant polycystic kidney disease. Increased fractional urate excretion is incorrect, as medullary cystic kidney disease is associated with hypouricosuria. Tamm–Horsfall protein is uromodulin. Tamm-Horsfall protein casts in the urine occur in myeloma cast nephropathy (by co-aggregation with Bence Jones proteins).

Hart TC, Gorry MC, Hart PS, et al. Mutations of the *UMOD* gene are responsible for medullary cystic kidney disease 2 and familial juvenile hyperuricaemic nephropathy. J Med Genet. 2002;39(12):882–92.

94. C. Plasma α-galactosidase A level.

The clinical picture is suggestive of classic Fabry (type 1) disease due to the age of onset and presence of angiokeratomas on the lower abdomen and thighs ('bathing trunk' distribution), alongside cardiac and renal pathology.

Late-onset Fabry (type 2) disease presents between the age of 30 and 70 years with renal and cardiac abnormalities. Fabry disease is an X-linked defect in the *GLA* gene, which codes for the enzyme α-galactosidase A. This enzyme usually breaks down globotriaosylceramide and glycosphingolipids in lysosomes; in Fabry disease, these are not broken down and accumulate in lysosomes across the body, with multisystem consequences. As it is X-linked, males are more severely affected and a diagnosis can be confirmed by low α-galactosidase A levels or absent α-galactosidase A. In females, α-galactosidase A may be normal, and so diagnosis requires gene analysis.

Management of Fabry disease involves enzyme replacement therapy to reduce the accumulation of globotriaosylceramide and glycosphingolipids in lysosomes, with subsequent slowing of complications and improvement in symptoms. Otherwise, treatment focusses on managing complications (e.g. nephrology input for progressive CKD and renal replacement therapy) and managing symptoms (e.g. analgesia for neuropathic pain). In addition, genetic counselling is recommended for all individuals (and their families) with Fabry disease.

Glucagon levels are usually assessed in cases of recurrent hypoglycaemia in the absence of diabetes mellitus. Peripheral leukocyte cystine levels are used in cystinosis. Serum galactose-1-phosphate levels are used in the diagnosis of galactosaemia. Serum caeruloplasmin levels are used in the diagnosis of Wilson's disease.

Zarate YA, Hopkin RJ. Fabry's disease. Lancet. 2008;372(9647):1427–35.

95. E. Penicillamine.

The clinical history of stone formation and significantly raised urinary cysteine level indicate a diagnosis of cystinuria. Cystinuria is an inherited metabolic disorder due to mutations in the *SLC3A1* and *SLC7A9* genes resulting in elevated amino acid levels (cysteine, arginine, lysine, and ornithine) in the urine due to impaired reabsorption. It is inherited in an autosomal recessive pattern.

Treatment aims to reduce urinary cysteine concentration. This can be done by:

- dilution (increased fluid intake)
- cysteine reduction (reduced consumption of animal protein)
- urinary alkalinization to reduce cysteine precipitation (potassium citrate or bicarbonate administration).

Genetic counselling is recommended to all individuals (and their families) with cystinuria.

If conservative measures fail, then thiol-containing drugs, such as tiopronin, can be used to promote cysteine solubility. If unavailable, D-penicillamine can be used as an alternative.

D-penicillamine increases the solubility of cysteine in the urine, reducing recurrent stone formation. Acetazolamide can, in theory, be used to promote urinary alkalinization, but it increases the risk of calcium phosphate stone formation and can adversely impact bone mineral density.

Servais A, Thomas K, Dello Strologo L, *et al.* Metabolic Nephropathy Workgroup of the European Reference Network for Rare Kidney Diseases (ERKNet) and eUROGEN. Cystinuria: clinical practice recommendation. Kidney Int. 2021;99(1):48–58.

Take-Home Messages

1. Non-visible haematuria over the age of 40, if symptomatic or with no evidence of renal disease, should be referred for cystoscopy.
2. In patients with diabetes and CKD, an alternative diagnosis can be considered if there is no evidence of diabetic retinopathy, a higher level of proteinuria, and a <5-year history of diabetes.

3. Common differentials for Glomerular causes of persistent non-visible haematuria are IgA nephropathy, Alport disease, and TBMN. In TBMN and Alport disease, electron microscopy shows thinning of the GBM (<200 nm).

4. TBMN is preferred over Alport disease if:
   a. no family history of kidney disease
   b. no clinical features of Alport disease (proteinuria, hearing loss, retinopathy, and lenticonus)
   c. no *COL4A5* mutation (if genetic testing is performed)
   d. absence of a 'lamellated' appearance of the GBM
   e. normal $\alpha 3$ and $\alpha 5$ type IV collagen units on immunofluorescence.
   Management of TBMN includes BP and proteinuria control.

5. Risk factors for IgAN progression are proteinuria, hypertension, MEST-C and impaired renal function. The mainstay of management includes RAS inhibition, BP control, and lifestyle optimization. Immunosuppression can be considered if IgAN presents as rapidly progressive, defined by >50% reduction in eGFR in 3 months.

6. Orthostatic proteinuria resolves in the recumbent position such as in sleep. A first morning void urine sample which yields no evidence of proteinuria confirms the diagnosis.

7. The TIN spectrum includes:
   a. rash
   b. arthralgia
   c. loin pain.
   Serum abnormalities may include:
   a. AKI
   b. eosinophilia
   c. thrombocytopenia
   d. anti-drug antibodies.
   Urine abnormalities may include:
   a. proteinuria
   b. haematuria
   c. leukocyturia (eosinophiluria).

8. On staining with Congo red, apple green birefringence is demonstrated under polarized light, characteristic of amyloidosis.

9. Exercise-induced haematuria is a benign condition that requires no further management. A single episode of haematuria warrants repeat testing for confirmation.

10. Membranous nephropathy has a higher risk of VTE due to a higher amount of proteinuria and possible association with underlying malignancy.

11. Features of Alport syndrome include:
    a. family history of kidney disease
    b. extra-renal manifestations (hearing loss, lenticonus)
    c. lamellation of the GBM on electron microscopy
    d. mutations of *COL4A5*.

12. TINU is TIN with uveitis; it affects young women commonly and steroids can be used for treatment.

13. Pamidronate causes FSGS. Other drugs causing secondary FSGS include opioids, anabolic steroids, calcineurin inhibitors, lithium, interferons, and sirolimus.

14. CKDu presentations include advanced kidney disease, muscle weakness and fatigue (caused by hypokalaemia), and sterile dysuria (caused by uric acid crystalluria). Electrolyte abnormalities characteristic of tubular dysfunction are present and include hypokalaemia, hyponatraemia, hypomagnesaemia, and hypophosphataemia.

15. MCKD, also known as autosomal dominant tubulointerstitial disease, develops due to mutations in:
    a. *UMOD* (commonest, codes for uromodulin and is associated with gout)
    b. *MUC1* (codes for mucin-1)
    c. *REN* (least common, codes for renin).

16. IgAN can only be diagnosed by biopsy, which will show predominant IgA +/− IgG and C3 mesangial deposits C1q and IgM will not be present.

17. Anti-phospholipase A2 receptor (PLA2R) antibodies are highly specific for primary MN (sensitivity 0.78, specificity 0.99). Anti-THSD7A antibodies are seen in 5% of primary MN cases.

18. CKD patients should be immunized against hepatitis B, Annual influenza and pneumococcal vaccines should also be offered.

19. Sodium phosphate is not recommended for bowel preparation in CKD due to the potential risk of severe AKI.

20. Risk factors for contrast-induced nephropathy include:
    a. CKD with eGFR <40 mL/min/1.73 m^2
    b. diabetes and eGFR <40 mL/min/1.73 m^2
    c. heart failure
    d. renal transplant
    e. age >75
    f. hypovolaemia
    g. high volume of contrast required
    h. arterial contrast with first-pass renal exposure.

21. Retroperitonal fibrosis can be associated with HLA-B27, other autoimmune diseases, and IgG4 disease. CRP and ESR can be elevated; patients can experience systemic symptoms and hydronephrosis can occur.

22. Anti-GBM disease usually presents as rapidly progressive glomerulonephritis, and almost two-thirds of patients have concurrent alveolar haemorrhage.

23. In vesicoureteric reflux, genetic patterns are heterogenous and no single gene locus or gene has been identified. There is an increased (but not quantifiable) risk of offspring being affected.

24. Fabry disease is an X-linked lysosomal disorder due to a gene defect encoding the α-galactosidase A enzyme.

25. Classic Fabry disease will lead to CKD (which contributes to hypertension), cardiac abnormalities (arrhythmia, hypertrophy), and an increased risk of a cerebrovascular event. In late-onset Fabry (type 2) disease, the patient presents with renal and cardiac abnormalities between the age of 30 and 70 years, with minimal other symptoms, due to residual enzyme activity.

26. Extra-renal manifestations of Alport syndrome include sensorineural deafness, ocular defects, and leiomyomatosis of the oesophagus and genitalia.

27. Renal impairment, medullary cysts, gout, and a family history together are suggestive of medullary cystic kidney disease, an autosomal dominant disorder.

28. In cystinuria, if conservative measures fail, thiol-containing drugs, such as tiopronin, can be used to promote cysteine solubility. D-penicillamine can be used as an alternative.

29. Tuberous sclerosis is characterized by:
    a. renal (angiomyolipomas, cysts)
    b. skin (facial angiofibromas, ungual or periungual fibromas, shagreen patches, and hypomelanotic macules)
    c. ocular (retinal hamartomas)
    d. central nervous system (epilepsy, giant cell astrocytomas)
    e. cardiac (rhabdomyomas)
    f. pulmonary (multifocal micronodular pneumocyte hyperplasia).

96. **A 63-year-old man was seen for follow-up in the renal clinic. He complained of feeling tired and lethargic, and a little less active than previously. He is known to have CKD stage 4, hypertension, and peripheral vascular disease, and takes clopidogrel, atorvastatin, ramipril, and bisoprolol.**

    On examination, his BP was 157/85 mmHg. The rest of the examination was unremarkable.

    Investigations:
haemoglobin	90 g/L (130–180)
haemoglobin (4 months ago)	97 g/L (130–180)
transferrin saturation	9% (20–50)
serum ferritin	35 µg/L (15–300)
eGFR	23 mL/min/1.73 m² (>60)

    What is the next best step in anaemia management?

    A. erythropoiesis-stimulating agent
    B. IV iron infusion
    C. oesophageal endoscopy
    D. oral iron
    E. stop clopidogrel

Best of Five MCQs for the European Specialty Examination in Nephrology. Shafi Malik, Oxford University Press.
© Oxford University Press 2024. DOI: 10.1093/oso/9780192844163.003.0009

97. **A 65-year-old man, who is on regular haemodialysis, is reviewed in the dialysis clinic for his monthly review. He undergoes three 4-hour dialysis sessions per week. His medications are darbepoetin alfa 80 μg weekly, felodipine 10 mg once daily, and alfacalcidol 250 ng once daily.**

    Investigations:
haemoglobin	89 g/L (130–180)
haemoglobin (3 months ago)	105 g/L (130–180)
serum ferritin	90 μg/L (15–300)
MCV	90 fL (80–96)
transferrin saturation	13% (20–50)
Kt/v	1.3
URR	70%
serum vitamin B_{12}	420 ng/L (160–760)
serum folate	2.50 μg/L (2.0–11.0)

    What is the next best step in management?

    A. increase the ESA dose
    B. IV iron
    C. oral folic acid
    D. oral iron
    E. switch darbepoetin to epoetin

98. **A 73-year-old man attended his regular follow-up clinic appointment. He has been feeling well and remained asymptomatic. He is active and enjoys working in his garden. His past history includes CKD stage 4 secondary to diabetic nephropathy, hypertension, and ischaemic stroke with no residual deficit. His medications include clopidogrel, atorvastatin, ramipril, linagliptin, and bisoprolol.**

    On examination, his BP was 137/82 mmHg. The rest of the examination was unremarkable.

    Investigations:
haemoglobin	98 g/L (130–180)
haemoglobin (4 months ago)	97 g/L (130–180)
transferrin saturation	31% (20–50)
serum ferritin	335 μg/L (15–300)
eGFR	23 mL/min/1.73 m² (>60)

    What is the most appropriate next step?

    A. erythropoiesis-stimulating agent
    B. IV iron
    C. no change
    D. oral iron
    E. stop clopidogrel

99. **A 72-year-old woman was reviewed in the haemodialysis clinic for routine follow-up. She reported feeling generally well, other than occasionally tired. Her medications include IV epoetin 3000 units thrice weekly on dialysis, IV iron sucrose 200 mg monthly, calcium acetate 1 g three times daily with meals, and alfacalcidol 250 ng once daily.**

On examination, apart from mild lower limb oedema, no other abnormality was detected.

Investigations:
haemoglobin   87 g/L (130–180)
serum ferritin   200 µg/L (15–300)
transferrin saturation   15% (20–50)
MCV   78 fL (80–96)
reticulocyte count   2% (0.5–2.4)

What is the most appropriate next step?

A. add oral iron
B. continue current treatment
C. increase ESA dose to 4000 units thrice weekly
D. increase the IV iron dose to 400 mg monthly
E. switch to another ESA

100. **A 75-year-old lady was seen in the low clearance clinic for regular follow-up. She has CKD stage 5–non-dialysis due to obstructive uropathy. In the clinic, she reported feeling well, other than tired. In the last 6 months, she was started on darbepoetin alfa 30 µg weekly, which was increased to 50 µg weekly to manage anaemia. Eight weeks prior, she was also given IV ferric carboxymaltose 1 g.**

Investigations:
eGFR   14 mL/min/1.73 m^2 (>60)
haemoglobin   85 g/L (130–180)
serum ferritin   450 µg/L (15–300)
transferrin saturation   25% (20–50)
MCV   89 fL (80–96)
reticulocyte count   2% (0.5–2.4)

What is the next best step?

A. add oral iron
B. another dose of IV iron
C. increase the dose of darbepoetin
D. switch to another ESA
E. upper GI endoscopy

101. A 45-year-old woman on haemodialysis via a tunnelled dialysis catheter is seen for routine follow-up. The patient has type 1 diabetes mellitus, diabetic retinopathy, peripheral neuropathy, and hypertension. In addition to antihypertensives, she is on epoetin alfa 3000 units thrice weekly.

On examination, her BP was 140/80 mmHg. She was pale and had mild bilateral lower limb swelling. The line exit site showed a yellow-coloured discharge.

Investigations:
haemoglobin	90 g/L (130–180)
serum ferritin	785 µg/L (15–300)
transferrin saturation	10% (20–50)
serum CRP	162 mg/L (<10)

What is the most appropriate next step in anaemia management?

A. blood transfusion
B. give IV iron
C. increase the ESA dose
D. postpone IV iron
E. switch to a long-acting ESA

102. A 45-year-old man on regular haemodiafiltration attended clinic for review. He is presently suspended from the transplant list due to low haemoglobin levels. He is currently on IV iron sucrose 400 µg once monthly and epoetin alfa 10,000 IU IV thrice weekly on dialysis.

His body weight is on target at 62 kg.

Investigations:
haemoglobin	87 g/L (130–180)
serum ferritin	600 µg/L (15–300)
transferrin saturation	30% (20–50)
URR	70
Kt/v	1.4

Which factor indicates resistance to ESA therapy?

A. dialysis adequacy
B. epoetin alfa dose
C. ferritin level
D. parathyroid hormone
E. transferrin saturation

103. **A 70-year-old man with focal segmental glomerulosclerosis attended the advanced kidney care clinic for routine follow-up. He is on maximum conservative care as per patient choice. In the clinic, he was asymptomatic, apart from some itching.**

> On examination, his BP was 130/80 mmHg and his heart rate was 75 beats/min. The patient had mild ankle swelling and there were scratch marks on his legs and arms.

Investigations:
serum creatinine   520 µmol/L (60–110)
serum adjusted calcium   2.1 mmol/L (2.20–2.60)
serum phosphate   2.1 mmol/L (0.80–1.45)
plasma parathyroid hormone   45 pmol/L (0.9–5.4)
serum 25-OH-cholecalciferol   50 nmol/L (50–120)

What is the next step in his MBD management?

A. alfacalcidol
B. calcium acetate
C. cinacalcet
D. cholecalciferol
E. sevelamer

104. **A 65-year-old man is reviewed in the dialysis clinic. He is on haemodialysis 3 times per weekly, with 4 hours each session of 4-hour duration, and is taking calcium acetate one tablet three times daily with meals.**

Investigations:
Kt/v   1.4
serum adjusted calcium   2.55 mmol/L (2.20–2.60)
serum phosphate   2.1 mmol/L (0.80–1.45)
plasma parathyroid hormone   10 pmol/L (0.9–5.4)

What is the next step in his MBD management?

A. add alfacalcidol
B. change to calcium carbonate
C. increase the dose of calcium acetate
D. increase the dialysis duration
E. switch to sevelamer

105. A 50-year-old man was reviewed on the haemodialysis unit. He had been on unit-based haemodialysis for 7 years. He had been treated with alfacalcidol 0.5 µg daily, and the dialysate calcium level has been maintained at 1.25 mmol/L. He had stopped taking calcium carbonate with meals 4 weeks previously.

Investigations:

serum adjusted calcium	2.50 mmol/L (2.20–2.60)
serum phosphate	2.1 mmol/L (0.80–1.45)
serum alkaline phosphatase	105 U/L (45–105)
plasma parathyroid hormone	60 pmol/L (0.9–5.4)
plasma parathyroid hormone (8 months ago)	55 pmol/L (0.9–5.4)

What is the most appropriate next step in management?

A. calcium acetate

B. cinacalcet

C. lanthanum carbonate

D. parathyroidectomy

E. paricalcitol

106. A 65-year-old man, who has been on dialysis for 9 years, is reviewed in clinic following monthly blood tests. Past history includes type 2 diabetes, ischaemic heart disease, and moderate to severe left ventricular systolic dysfunction. He was taking calcium acetate 2 g three times daily and alfacalcidol 1 µg daily.

Investigations:

transferrin saturation	22% (20–50)
serum adjusted calcium	2.50 mmol/L (2.20–2.60)
serum phosphate	1.6 mmol/L (0.80–1.45)
serum alkaline phosphatase	160 U/L (45–105)
plasma parathyroid hormone	112 pmol/L (0.9–5.4)

What is the most appropriate next step?

A. increase the dose of calcium acetate

B. increase the dose of oral alfacalcidol

C. refer for parathyroidectomy

D. start a calcimimetic

E. start IV alfacalcidol

107. **A 32-year-old man on haemodialysis was admitted following a low-impact hip fracture. He has had CKD since childhood secondary to haemolytic uraemic syndrome, and has had two failed renal transplants. Treatment adherence has been poor over the years. Current medications include cinacalcet 120 mg once daily, sevelamer carbonate 800 mg three times daily, and IV alfacalcidol.**

Investigations:
serum adjusted calcium   2.70 mmol/L (2.20–2.60)
serum phosphate   2.27 mmol/L (0.80–1.45)
serum alkaline phosphatase   535 U/L (45–105)
plasma parathyroid hormone   935 pmol/L (0.9–5.4)

What is the next best management step?

A. add lanthanum carbonate
B. increase the dose of cinacalcet
C. parathyroidectomy
D. reduce the dose of alfacalcidol
E. switch to IV calcimimetic

108. **A 75-year-old man on regular haemodialysis attended the haemodialysis clinic. He had ESRD due to diabetic nephropathy. He had a background of type 2 diabetes mellitus, ischaemic heart disease, diabetic retinopathy, and diabetic neuropathy.**

You discussed with him the recent monthly blood results, with a certain emphasis on his mineral bone findings.

Investigations:
Kt/v   1.4
serum adjusted calcium   2.47 mmol/L (2.20–2.60)
serum phosphate   1.88 mmol/L (0.80–1.45)
serum alkaline phosphatase   40 U/L (45–105)
plasma parathyroid hormone   6.6 pmol/L (0.9–5.4)

Which histological type of mineral bone disease is this man most likely to have?

A. adynamic bone disease
B. mixed uraemic bone disease
C. osteitis fibrosa cystica
D. osteomalacia
E. osteoporosis

109. **A 68-year-old lady attended her regular follow-up. She was asymptomatic and reported feeling well. She has a past history of CKD stage 3, hypothyroidism, hypertension, gout, and vitamin B12 deficiency. She is on atorvastatin, amlodipine, levothyroxine, vitamin B12, allopurinol, and ferrous fumarate.**

Investigations:
eGFR	31 mL/min/1.73 m^2 (>60)
serum adjusted calcium	2.80 mmol/L (2.20–2.60)
serum phosphate	1.15 mmol/L (0.80–1.45)
plasma parathyroid hormone	128 pmol/L (0.9–5.4)
serum 25-OH-cholecalciferol	50 nmol/L (50–120)

What is the most likely diagnosis?

A. hypovitaminosis D

B. primary hyperparathyroidism

C. resistant secondary hyperparathyroidism

D. secondary hyperparathyroidism

E. tertiary hyperparathyroidism

110. **A 55-year-old lady attended the low clearance clinic for a routine review. She had CKD stage 4 due to diabetic nephropathy.**

On examination, her BP was 130/80 mmHg. Examination was otherwise unremarkable.

Investigations:
eGFR	18 mL/min/1.73 m^2 (>60)
serum adjusted calcium	2.20 mmol/L (2.20–2.60)
serum phosphate	1.5 mmol/L (0.80–1.45)
plasma parathyroid hormone	10.5 pmol/L (0.9–5.4)

How frequent should parathyroid hormone be monitored?

A. 18–24 months

B. 4–6 months

C. 6–12 months

D. monthly

E. quarterly

96. D. Oral iron.

This anaemic patient with CKD stage 4 has an absolute iron deficiency, as his ferritin level is <100 ng/mL and transferrin saturation is 9%. Starting erythropoietin treatment in this iron-deficient patient will not manage his iron deficiency. According to guidance from NICE, therapy with an ESA should not be started in the presence of absolute iron deficiency without also managing the iron deficiency. Furthermore, in non-dialysis CKD patients, a trial of oral iron should be considered before offering IV iron therapy. If the patients are intolerant of oral iron or target haemoglobin levels are not achieved within 3 months, then IV iron is offered. In absolute iron deficiency anaemia, treatment with iron is recommended prior to endoscopic examination.

National Institute for Health and Care Excellence (2021). Chronic kidney disease: assessment and management. NICE guideline [NG203]. Available from: https://www.nice.org.uk/guidance/ng203 (see anaemia management section).

Snook J, Bhala N, Beales ILP, et al. British Society of Gastroenterology guidelines for the management of iron deficiency anaemia in adults. Gut. 2021;70:2030–51.

97. B. IV iron.

This patient is iron-deficient. Increasing the ESA dose is of little value in the presence of iron deficiency. Switching erythropoietin will not help either for the same reason. In dialysis patients, IV iron is better tolerated and more efficacious than oral iron. The PIVOTAL trial showed high dose IV iron is better than low-dose IV iron.

Macdougall IC, White C, Anker SD, et al.; PIVOTAL Investigators and Committees. Intravenous iron in patients undergoing maintenance hemodialysis. N Engl J Med. 2019;380(5):447–58.

The Renal Association (2017, updated 2020). Clinical practice guideline anaemia of chronic kidney disease. Available from: https://ukkidney.org/sites/renal.org/files/Updated-130220-Anaemia-of-Chronic-Kidney-Disease-1-1.pdf

98. C. No change.

This patient is anaemic. He has good iron stores, so both choices of oral and IV iron are not indicated. Also, the haemoglobin level is stable, with no evidence of blood loss, which makes stopping clopidogrel inappropriate. According to KDIGO anaemia guidelines, therapy with an ESA should be started in symptomatic patients. As this patient is asymptomatic with stable haemoglobin levels, no change is recommended in his current treatment.

Kidney Disease: Improving Global Outcomes (KDIGO) Anemia Work Group. KDIGO clinical practice guideline for anemia in chronic kidney disease. Kidney Int (Suppl). 2012;2:279–335.

99. D. Increase the IV iron dose to 400 mg monthly.

This patient has iron deficiency anaemia, as transferrin saturation is 15%. Increasing the ESA dose, or switching to another ESA, will not help in managing the patient's anaemia. The Renal Association guidelines recommend for haemodialysis patients high-dose IV iron sucrose 400 mg every month (or equivalent) to be given, unless ferritin levels are >700 µg/L, or transferrin saturation >40%, based on the PIVOTAL trial.

Macdougall IC, White C, Anker SD, et al.; PIVOTAL Investigators and Committees. Intravenous iron in patients undergoing maintenance hemodialysis. N Engl J Med. 2019;380(5):447–58.

The Renal Association (2017, updated 2020). Clinical practice guideline anaemia of chronic kidney disease. Available from: https://ukkidney.org/health-professionals/information-resources/uk-eckd-guide/anaemia

100. C. Increase the dose of darbepoetin.

This lady has satisfactory iron stores. Both the MCV and reticulocyte count are normal. Increasing the ESA dose would be the best step. It is recommended to increase the dose by 25%. There is no evidence of blood loss.

Guedes M, Robinson BM, Obrador G, Tong A, Pisoni RL, Pecoits-Filho R. Management of anemia in nondialysis chronic kidney disease: current recommendations, real-world practice, and patient perspectives. Kidney360. 2020;1(8):855–62.

101. D. Postpone IV iron.

This patient most likely has tunnelled line infection, in addition to iron deficiency anaemia. Ferritin is an inflammatory marker. Some studies have shown an increase in mortality and infection due to oxidative stress when IV iron is given during active infection. This could also be due to IV iron increasing the levels of circulating non-transferrin-bound iron, which may promote pathogenic growth. In the presence of iron deficiency, increasing or changing the dose of erythropoietin will be less effective in managing anaemia.

Shah AA, Donovan K, Seeley C, et al. Risk of infection associated with administration of intravenous iron: a systematic review and meta-analysis. JAMA Netw Open. 2021;4(11):e2133935.

102. B. Epoetin alfa dose.

This case scenario discusses erythropoietin (EPO) resistance. This patient is on an IV EPO dose of >450 IU/kg per week. Inadequate response ('resistance') to therapy with an ESA is defined as failure to reach the target haemoglobin level despite a subcutaneous epoetin alfa dose of >300 IU/kg per week, or an IV epoetin alfa dose of 450 IU/kg per week, or a darbepoetin dose of >1.5 µg/kg per week. Hyporesponsive patients who are iron-replete should be screened clinically and by investigation for other common causes of anaemia.

Batchelor EK, Kapitsinou P, Pergola PE, Kovesdy CP, Jalal DI. Iron deficiency in chronic kidney disease: updates on pathophysiology, diagnosis, and treatment. J Am Soc Nephrol. 2020;31(3):456–68.

103. B. Calcium acetate.

This patient has hyperphosphataemia and secondary hyperparathyroidism. The vitamin D level is satisfactory, while the target vitamin D level in CKD patients is >30 nmol/L. This patient has hyperphosphataemia, which alfacalcidol and cholecalciferol will worsen. As the calcium level is lower than normal, cinacalcet is not a good choice. A calcium-based binder would be appropriate when the serum calcium level is low normal. Moreover, in a patient being managed conservatively, a calcium-based binder would be reasonable. This is also in keeping with guidelines from NICE which recommend calcium-based binders as the first choice.

Burton JO, Goldsmith DJ, Ruddock N, *et al.* Renal Association commentary on the KDIGO (2017) clinical practice guideline update for the diagnosis, evaluation, prevention, and treatment of CKD-MBD. BMC Nephrol. 2018;19:240.

National Institute for Health and Care Excellence (2021). Chronic kidney disease: assessment and management. NICE guideline [NG203]. Available from: https://www.nice.org.uk/guidance/ng203

104. E. Switch to sevelamer.

This case scenario describes a haemodialysis patient with adequate dialysis parameters. This patient has hyperphosphataemia and his corrected calcium level is high normal. Also, parathyroid hormone (PTH) is suppressed below the target level, which is 2–9 times the upper limit of normal. In this case, adding alfacalcidol would cause further PTH suppression and a rise in the phosphate level (alfacalcidol increases both serum calcium and phosphate levels). Changing to calcium carbonate may worsen serum calcium and PTH levels. There is no indication to increase the duration of dialysis. Increasing the dose of calcium acetate will worsen hypercalcaemia and PTH suppression.

Spoendlin J, Paik JM, Tsacogianis T, Kim SC, Schneeweiss S, Desai RJ. Cardiovascular outcomes of calcium-free vs calcium-based phosphate binders in patients 65 years or older with end-stage renal disease requiring hemodialysis. JAMA Intern Med. 2019;179(6):741–9.

105. C. Lanthanum carbonate.

This patient has hyperphosphataemia and hyperparathyroidism. Adding calcium acetate or increasing the alfacalcidol dose will likely lead to hypercalcaemia, carrying a greater risk of vascular calcification. Adding cinacalcet or parathyroidectomy will manage hyperparathyroidism, but not hyperphosphataemia. Paricalcitol would be indicated if the patient was optimized on a phosphate binder. The best choice would be using a non-calcium based binder.

Kidney Disease: Improving Global Outcomes (KDIGO) CKD–MBD Update Work Group. KDIGO 2017 Clinical practice guideline update for the diagnosis, evaluation, prevention, and treatment of chronic kidney disease–mineral and bone disorder (CKD–MBD). Kidney Int Suppl. 2017;7:1–59.

106. D. Start a calcimimetic.

This haemodialysis patient has hyperparathyroidism and at the same time, he has a corrected calcium level in the upper limit of normal. He is on calcium acetate 2 g three times daily and alfacalcidol 1 µg daily. Increasing the dose of calcium acetate or oral alfacalcidol, or starting IV alfacalcidol, will lead to further hypercalcaemia. Parathyroidectomy is not a suitable choice for a patient with moderate left ventricular systolic dysfunction. So the best action in this case is to use cinacalcet to inhibit parathyroid hormone secretion and at the same time, it may reduce serum calcium level.

The mechanism of action of cinacalcet is that of a calcimimetic which acts on calcium-sensing receptors. It simulates the effect of calcium on calcium receptors in the parathyroid gland. This gives the parathyroid gland the impression that there is a higher calcium level in blood, which inhibits secretion of parathyroid hormone.

National Institute for Health and Care Excellence (2007). Cinacalcet for the treatment of secondary hyperparathyroidism in patients with end-stage renal disease on maintenance dialysis therapy. Technology appraisal guidance [TA117]. Available from: https://www.nice.org.uk/guidance/ta117

107. C. Parathyroidectomy.

This haemodialysis patient has tertiary hyperparathyroidism. He has very high parathyroid hormone level with hypercalcaemia and hyperphosphataemia with high bone turnover indicated by high alkaline phosphatase level. This patient also had a low impact hip fracture suggesting bone fragility meaning his hyperparathyroidism should be treated urgently. As the patient is suitable for operative intervention, parathyroidectomy would be the best choice according to the NICE guidelines which suggest referral for parathyroidectomy as long as they are fit and suitable for the procedure. Switch to IV calcimimetic is not indicated as the patient is tolerating oral cinacalcet. Also, increasing cinacalcet in this scenario will not achieve the required effect.

National Institute for Health and Care Excellence (2007). Cinacalcet for the treatment of secondary hyperparathyroidism in patients with end-stage renal disease on maintenance dialysis therapy. Technology guidance appraisal. Available from: https://www.nice.org.uk/guidance/ta117/resources/cin acalcet-for-the-treatment-of-secondary-hyperparathyroidism-in-patients-with-endstage-renal-disease-on-maintenance-dialysis-therapy-pdf-82598077917637

National Institute for Health and Care Excellence (2017). Etelcalcetide for treating secondary hyperparathyroidism. Technology appraisal guidance [TA448]. Available from: https://www.nice.org.uk/guidance/ta448

108. A. Adynamic bone disease.

TH is oversuppressed in this case. In haemodialysis patients, the target parathyroid hormone level is 2–9 times the upper limit of normal. Additionally, this man has low alkaline phosphatase level, reflecting low bone turnover, likely due to adynamic bone disease. Serum parathyroid hormone level over twice the upper limit of normal, together with low alkaline phosphatase level and the patient being diabetic, all point towards this diagnosis.

Martin KJ, Floege J, Ketteler M. Bone and mineral disorders in chronic kidney disease. In: J Feehally, J Floege, M Tonelli, eds. *Comprehensive Clinical Nephrology*, 6th edition. St Louis, MO: Elsevier, 2019; pp. 979–95.

109. B. Primary hyperparathyroidism.

This lady has CKD stage 3B with hypercalcaemia and hyperparathyroidism. Vitamin D level is satisfactory. Therefore, the high parathyroid hormone level is not due to hypovitaminosis D. The criteria for secondary or tertiary hyperparathyroidism are not fulfilled.

Hyder R, Sprague SM. Secondary hyperparathyroidism in a patient with CKD. Clin J Am Soc Nephrol. 2020;15(7):1041–3.

110. C. 6–12 months.

The frequency of testing of hyperparathyroidism differs according to the CKD stage. According to the UK Renal Association guidelines, in CKD stage 4, parathyroid hormone levels should be tested at an interval of 6–12 months.

Kidney Disease: Improving Global Outcomes (KDIGO) CKD-MBD Update Work Group. KDIGO 2017 clinical practice guideline update for the diagnosis, evaluation, prevention, and treatment of chronic kidney disease–mineral and bone disorder (CKD-MBD). Kidney Int Suppl. 2017;7(1):1–59.

Take-Home Messages

1. Peritubular capillary cells secrete EPO. Lack of secretion leads to renal anaemia in CKD patients.
2. Renal anaemia is more evident in severe CKD with eGFR <30 mL/min. Anaemia in CKD patients with eGFR >30 mL/min should be investigated for other causes of anaemia, including age-matched cancer.

3. Iron-deficient CKD non-dialysis patients should be managed with oral iron, followed by iron infusion if non-responsive. Iron-deficient CKD dialysis patients are managed with IV iron infusion.

4. The PIVOTAL trial showed that proactive use of 400-mg IV iron infusion monthly in haemodialysis patients (cut-off for ferritin level 700 μg/L, transferrin saturation 40%) is associated with fewer cardiovascular events, compared to use of 200-mg IV infusion monthly.

5. The target haemoglobin level in patients treated with ESAs is 100–120 g/L. Haemoglobin levels of >130 g/L carry a risk of thrombosis and stroke.

6. In cases of EPO unresponsiveness, causes for refractoriness include iron deficiency, vitamin B12 deficiency, folate deficiency, infection, underdialysis, poor compliance, blood loss, and hyperparathyroidism, as well as haematological disorders such as bone marrow diseases, sickle cell disease, and anti-EPO antibodies causing pure red cell aplasia.

7. Management of CKD-MBD involves low-phosphate diet, use of phosphate binders, and appropriate use of vitamin D analogues.

8. For dietary restriction, it is recommended to restrict phosphorus intake to 600–900 mg/day.

9. Phosphate binders reduce enteric absorption of ingested phosphorus. Calcium-based binders (calcium carbonate or calcium acetate) are frequently used in CKD patients. Non-calcium binders, such as sevelamer hydrochloride or carbonate, lanthanum carbonate, and sucroferric oxyhydroxide (iron-based binder), are not approved for use in pre-dialysis CKD.

10. Limiting the amount of daily elemental calcium intake to no more than 2000 mg/day is recommended due to the risk of increased calcium loading and vascular calcification.

11. The target level of vitamin D in CKD patients is >30 ng/mL. Cholecalciferol (vitamin D3) or ergocalciferol (vitamin D2) can be used for vitamin D replacement. Vitamin D replacement should be postponed in patients with hypercalcaemia or hyperphosphataemia.

12. Active vitamin D and vitamin D analogues (1,25-dihydroxycholecalciferol) reduce parathyroid hormone production and secretion through a negative feedback mechanism.

13. Secondary hyperparathyroidism is managed with vitamin D analogues (e.g. alfacalcidol) or a calcimimetic (e.g. cinacalcet), with parathyroidectomy recommended for patients fit for surgery.

111. **A 52-year-old man with type 2 diabetes and CKD is seen for follow-up. At his last review 3 months ago, he had a GFR of 48 mL/min/1.73 m² and a urinary albumin:creatinine ratio of 79 mg/mmol.**

What is the recommended haemoglobin A_{1c} target in this patient?

   A. ≤7.0%
   B. ≤6.5%
   C. <7.0% to <8.0%
   D. <6.5% to <8.0%
   E. ≤8.0%

112. **A 63-year-old lady with CKD stage G4 A3 comes to see you in clinic. Her BP was 141/87 mmHg and she had a trace of ankle oedema. She takes ramipril 10 mg once daily.**

   She is keen to avoid taking additional tablets and asks you if there are any dietary modifications that she can try.

   What would be your recommendation?

   A. aim for sodium restriction of <1.5 g/day
   B. aim for sodium restriction of <2.4 g/day
   C. aim for sodium restriction of <2 g/day
   D. dietary sodium restriction is largely ineffective, prescribe amlodipine
   E. dietary sodium restriction is largely ineffective, prescribe bendroflumethiazide

Best of Five MCQs for the European Specialty Examination in Nephrology. Shafi Malik, Oxford University Press.
© Oxford University Press 2024. DOI: 10.1093/oso/9780192844163.003.0011

113. Regarding diabetes and non-dialysis-dependent CKD, which one of the following statements is true?

A. an angiotensin-converting enzyme inhibitor or angiotensin receptor blocker should be used in adults with a urine albumin excretion of <30 mg per 24 hours

B. in patients with a urine albumin excretion <30 mg per 24 hours, the treatment target for BP is ≤140 mmHg systolic and ≤90 mmHg diastolic

C. in patients with a urine albumin excretion <30 mg per 24 hours, the treatment target for BP is ≤130 mmHg systolic and ≤80 mmHg diastolic

D. in patients with a urine albumin excretion >30 mg per 24 hours, the treatment target for BP is ≤140 mmHg systolic and ≤90 mmHg diastolic

E. all statements are false

114. A 47-year-old man is referred to the renal clinic by his GP for management of CKD and proteinuria. He is known to have type 2 diabetes and hypertension, and was taking sitagliptin and bisoprolol.

On examination, he was euvolaemic and his BP was 130/76 mmHg.

Investigations:
serum creatinine   120 µmol/L (60–110)
eGFR   65 mL/min/1.73 m² (>60)
urine albumin:creatinine ratio   45 mg/mmol (<2.5)

You consider starting an SGLT2i, and as part of shared decision-making, the patient asks for facts related to the drug.

Which statement is incorrect?

A. a falling eGFR is an indication to stop SGLT2i therapy

B. an SGLT2i should be suspended during periods of prolonged fasting, for surgery, or during an acute intercurrent illness

C. once initiated, it is reasonable to continue an SGLT2i if the eGFR falls below 30 mL/min/1.73 m²

D. for patients with CKD with an eGFR ≤30 mL/min/1.73 m², an SGLT2i should be used in conjunction with metformin

E. patients with type 2 diabetes, CKD, and an eGFR ≤30 mL/min/1.73 m² should be treated with an SGLT2i

115. **A 45-year-old man with type 2 diabetes attends the CKD clinic. He takes metformin 1 g twice a day and ramipril 10 mg once a day. He had some blood and urine tests done last week in preparation for his clinic visit.**

Investigations:

serum urea	9.8 mmol/L (2.5–7.0)
serum creatinine	170 μmol/L (60–110)
eGFR	41 mL/min/1.73 m^2 (>60)
urine albumin:creatinine ratio	154 mg/mmol (<2.5)
haemoglobin A$_{1c}$	50 mmol/mol (20–42)

Which treatment step would you initiate?

A. canagliflozin 300 mg once a day

B. dapagliflozin 10 mg once a day

C. empagliflozin 5 mg once a day

D. gliclazide 80 mg once a day

E. make no changes to his treatment

116. **Regarding the mechanism of action of SGLT2i, which of the following statements is true?**

A. activates peroxisome proliferator-activated receptor gamma, altering the transcription of genes encoding glucose and lipid metabolism

B. binds to an ATP-dependent K$^+$ channel on the cell membranes of pancreatic β-cells, leading to an increase in endogenous insulin production

C. inhibits active reverse co-transport of sodium and glucose on the luminal surface of the S1 segment of the proximal renal tubule

D. inhibits degradation of incretins, glucagon-like peptide-1, and glucose-dependent insulinotropic peptide

E. stimulates release of insulin from the pancreatic islet cells in response to a glucose load, delays gastric emptying, and suppresses appetite stimulation via the central nervous system

117. **A 75-year-old woman with COPD, type 2 diabetes, and CKD stage 3b A2 is started on losartan 50 mg once a day by her GP. She was originally taking ramipril 5 mg but developed an irritating dry cough, and requested an alternative.**

On examination, her BP was 119/70 mmHg.

Investigations:
(2 months ago)

serum urea	7.6 mmol/L (2.5–7.0)
serum creatinine	136 μmol/L (60–110)
eGFR	34 mL/min/1.73 m² (>60)

(latest)

serum urea	9.2 mmol/L (2.5–7.0)
serum creatinine	181 μmol/L (60–110)
eGFR	25 mL/min/1.73 m² (>60)

What is the most appropriate next step?

A. continue losartan
B. reduce losartan by 50%
C. stop losartan
D. switch to amlodipine
E. switch to ramipril

118. **A 55-year-old man with proteinuric CKD due to diabetic nephropathy is seen in the renal clinic for follow-up. He was taking ramipril 5 mg once a day, amlodipine 10 mg once a day, sodium bicarbonate 1000 mg twice a day, and canagliflozin 100 mg once a day.**

On examination, his BP was 161/87 mmHg.

Investigations:

serum creatinine	185 μmol/L (60–110)
serum potassium	6.1 mmol/L (3.5–4.9)
serum bicarbonate	22 mmol/L (20–28)
urine albumin:creatinine ratio	478 mg/mmol (<2.5)

What is the next best step in management?

A. stop ramipril
B. start sodium zirconium cyclosilicate
C. refer to dietician
D. reduce ramipril dose by 50%
E. start furosemide

119. Regarding glucagon-like peptide-1 receptor agonists, which of the following statements is true?

A. the effect of incretin is increased in patients with T2DM

B. GLP-1 RA should be used in the place of SGLT2i if a patient's glycaemic target has not been met

C. in a meta-analysis, GLP-1 RA resulted in a 17% reduction in a composite kidney outcome, mainly due to a reduction in urine albumin excretion

D. in a meta-analysis, GLP-1 RA resulted in no significant reduction in major adverse cardiovascular events, death from cardiovascular causes, or fatal or non-fatal stroke

E. the risk of hypoglycaemia is low when a GLP-1 RA is used alongside insulin

120. A 45-year-old man attends the CKD clinic. He is known to have type 2 diabetes and CKD stage 3b A3. He is struggling to lose weight and has also seen a dietician. He reports increasing shortness of breath on exertion. Current medications include metformin, gliclazide, ramipril, amlodipine, sitagliptin, and canagliflozin. His home capillary blood glucose readings are 10–15 mmol/L.

On examination, there was moderate bilateral lower limb oedema. His BP was 151/94 mmHg, weight 96 kg, and BMI 33.2 kg/m².

Investigations:
(3 months ago)

eGFR	34 mL/min/1.73 m² (>60)
urine albumin:creatinine ratio	521 mg/mmol (<2.5)
haemoglobin A1c	8.1 mmol/mol (20–42)

(Latest)

eGFR	32 mL/min/1.73 m² (>60)
urine albumin:creatinine ratio	601 mg/mmol (<2.5)
haemoglobin A1c	7.9 mmol/mol (20–42)

What is the next most appropriate step in his management?

A. start insulin degludec

B. start insulin degludec with liraglutide

C. start liraglutide and stop metformin

D. start liraglutide, and stop sitagliptin and gliclazide

E. start liraglutide, stop sitagliptin, and reduce gliclazide

111. D. <6.5% to <8.0%.

The 2020 KDIGO Clinical Practice Guideline for Diabetes Management in CKD recommends an individualized HbA1c target ranging from <6.5% to <8.0% in patients with diabetes and non-dialysis-dependent CKD. This considers individual patient factors such as the need for prevention of micro- and macrovascular complications (e.g. in younger patients with early CKD), the risk of hypoglycaemia, other comorbidities, use of anti-hyperglycaemic agents, severity of CKD, and life expectancy. Answer A is the recommended target HbA1c for non-CKD patients who are treated with more than one anti-hyperglycaemic agent as per the National Institute for Health and Care Excellence. Answer B is the target for non-CKD patients with diabetes managed by either diet and lifestyle and/or a combination of diet and lifestyle and a single agent not associated with hypoglycaemia. The accuracy of HbA1c is reduced in patients with an eGFR <30 mL/min/1.73 m^2 due to shortened erythrocyte lifespan, producing lower values, as well as treatment with erythropoiesis-stimulating agents. As such, HbA1c values in patients with advanced CKD should be interpreted within these constraints.

Kidney Disease: Improving Global Outcomes (KDIGO) Diabetes Work Group. KDIGO 2020 Clinical Practice Guideline for Diabetes Management in Chronic Kidney Disease. Kidney Int. 2020;98(4S):S1–115.

112. C. Aim for sodium restriction of <2 g/day.

The 2020 KDIGO Clinical Practice Guideline for Diabetes Management in CKD recommends that sodium intake should be <2 g/day, equivalent to <90 mmol of sodium per day or <5 g of sodium chloride per day. Dietary sodium restriction lowers BP and is associated with improved cardiovascular outcomes in both patients with and those without CKD. However, patients with CKD are salt-sensitive and exhibit impaired homeostasis in regulating BP and extracellular volume status in the context of high salt intake. Therefore, restriction of dietary salt may have beneficial effects in both lowering BP and improving the volume status of the patient. Some studies have also shown that reducing sodium intake might enhance the action of diuretics and RAS blockade in CKD patients. Patients, such as the one described in this question, who are keen to avoid an increased pill burden are more likely to be motivated by this recommendation and tolerate the dietary changes needed, including those with reduced palatability. The 2021 KDIGO Clinical Practice Guideline for the Management of Blood Pressure in CKD suggests that patients undertake moderate-intensity physical activity for a total of 150 minutes per week, based on physical or cardiovascular tolerance. Of note, the 2021 KDIGO Blood Pressure Guideline now recommends adults with hypertension and CKD should be treated to a tighter target systolic BP of <120 mmHg (previously ≤130/80 mmHg for diabetic and non-diabetic adults with CKD with urine albumin excretion of >30 mg per 24 hours). However, the applicability of this target in people with diabetic kidney disease is debated. This target may not be achievable in this patient with lifestyle modification alone, and more than one antihypertensive agent may be required after incorporation of dietary salt restriction and regular physical exercise.

Kidney Disease: Improving Global Outcomes (KDIGO) Blood Pressure Work Group. KDIGO 2012 Clinical Practice Guideline for the Management of Blood Pressure in Chronic Kidney Disease. Kidney Int Suppl. 2012;2(5):337–414.

Kidney Disease: Improving Global Outcomes (KDIGO) Blood Pressure Work Group. KDIGO 2021 Clinical Practice Guideline for the Management of Blood Pressure in Chronic Kidney Disease. Kidney Int Suppl. 2021;99(3S):S1–87.

113. E. All statements are false.

The answers A to D relate to the previous KDIGO 2012 guidelines. The KDIGO 2021 Clinical Practice Guideline for the Management of Blood Pressure in CKD recommends a target systolic BP of <120 mmHg. The previous KDIGO 2012 guideline, suggesting a lower BP target for patients with albuminuria (≤130/80 mmHg), compared to those without, has been removed, based on inconclusive evidence that a lower BP target in the presence of proteinuria reduces the risk of progression to ESRD and there was no discernible effect modification with respect to proteinuria. Based on up-to-date evidence of cardiovascular and survival outcomes, the adoption of a new, lower systolic BP target for all CKD patients means that separate targets for albuminuria are not required. There is a wide base of evidence that use of RAS inhibitors in patients with diabetes and CKD reduces the risk of progression of CKD in relation to the development of severely increased albuminuria or doubling of serum creatinine(see table 6.1). The applicability of this new BP target is less certain in those with diabetic kidney disease, as the recommendation is based on SPRINT (Systolic Blood Pressure Intervention Trial), which did not include patients with diabetes. Furthermore, the ACCORD trial did not show any benefit of intensive BP control (systolic BP <120 mmHg), in terms of cardiovascular outcomes, excepting non-fatal stroke, in diabetics, compared to standard BP control (systolic BP <140 mmHg). In patients with diabetes, KDIGO recommends starting a RAS inhibitors in the presence of hypertension, CKD, and moderately to severely increased albuminuria (G1–4, A2 and A3). These medications should be titrated to the

Table 6.1 Different formulations of ACEis and ARBs

Drug		Starting dose	Maximum daily dose	Kidney impairment
ACE inhibitors	Benazepril	10 mg once daily	80 mg	CrCl ≥ 30 mL/min: no dosage adjustment needed CrCl <30 mL/min: reduce initial dose to 5 mg PO once daily for adults. Parent compound not removed by haemodialysis
	Captopril	12.5–25 mg 2–3 times daily	Usually 50 mg three times daily (may go up to 450 mg/day)	The half-life is increased in patients with renal impairment CrCl 10–50 mL/min: administer 75% of normal dose every 12–18 hours CrCl <10 mL/min: administer 50% of normal dose every 24 hours. Haemodialysis: administer after dialysis; about 40% of the drug is removed by haemodialysis

(continued)

Table 6.1 Continued

Drug		Starting dose	Maximum daily dose	Kidney impairment
	Enalapril	5 mg once daily	40 mg	CrCl ≤30 mL/min: in adult patients, reduce the initial dose to 2.5 mg PO once daily 2.5 mg PO after haemodialysis on dialysis days; dosage on non-dialysis days should be adjusted based on clinical response
	Fosinopril	10 mg once daily	80 mg	No dosage adjustment necessary Poorly removed by haemodialysis
	Lisinopril	10 mg once daily	40 mg	CrCl 10–30 mL/min: reduce the initial recommended dose by 50% for adults. Max: 40 mg/day CrCl <10 mL/min: reduce initial dosage to 2.5 mg PO once daily. Max: 40 mg/day
	Perindopril	2 mg once daily	8 mg	Use is not recommended when CrCl <30 mL/min Perindopril and its metabolites are removed by haemodialysis
	Quinapril	10 mg once daily	80 mg	CrCl 61–89 mL/min: start at 10 mg once daily CrCl 30–60 mL/min: start at 5 mg once daily CrCl 10–29 mL/min: start at 2.5 mg once daily CrCl <10 mL/min: insufficient data for dosage recommendation About 12% of parent compound removed by haemodialysis
	Ramipril	2.5 mg once daily	20 mg	Administer 25% of normal dose when CrCl <40 mL/min Minimally removed by haemodialysis
	Trandolapril	1 mg once daily	4 mg	CrCl <30 mL/min: reduce initial dose to 0.5 mg/day
Angiotensin receptor blockers	Azilsartan	20–80 mg once daily	80 mg	Dose adjustment is not required in patients with mild to severe renal impairment or renal failure
	Candesartan	16 mg once daily	32 mg	In patients with CrCl <30 mL/min, AUC and Cmax were approximately doubled with repeated dosing Not removed by haemodialysis
	Irbesartan	150 mg once daily	300 mg	No dosage adjustment necessary Not removed by haemodialysis
	Losartan	50 mg once daily	100 mg	No dosage adjustment necessary Not removed by haemodialysis
	Olmesartan	20 mg once daily	40 mg	AUC is increased 3-fold in patients with CrCl <20 mL/min No initial dosage adjustment is recommended for patients with moderate to marked renal impairment (CrCl <40 mL/min) Has not been studied in dialysis patients

Table 6.1 Continued

Drug		Starting dose	Maximum daily dose	Kidney impairment
	Telmisartan	40 mg once daily	80 mg	No dosage adjustment necessary Not removed by haemodialysis
	Valsartan	80 mg once daily	320 mg	No dosage adjustment available for CrCl <30 mL/min—to use with caution Not removed significantly by haemodialysis

Abbreviations: ACEi, angiotensin-converting enzyme inhibitor(s); ARB, angiotensin II receptor blocker; AUC, area under the curve; Cmax, maximum or peak concentration; CrCl, creatinine clearance; GFR, glomerular filtration rate.
Reproduced with permission from KDIGO 2020 Clinical Practice Guideline for Diabetes Management in Chronic Kidney Disease. *Kidney International*, Vol 98. Issue 45. 2020.

highest recommended dose that is tolerated. Similar recommendations apply for patients without diabetes with moderately (A2) and severely increased albuminuria (A3).

ACCORD Study Group. Effects of intensive blood-pressure control in type 2 diabetes mellitus. N Engl J Med. 2010;362:1575–85.

SPRINT Research Group. A randomized trial of intensive versus standard blood-pressure control. N Engl J Med. 2015;373:2103–16.

114. A. A falling eGFR is an indication to stop SGLT2i therapy.

A reversible decrease in eGFR was observed in landmark RCTs in participants who were treated with SGLT2i. However, since SGLT2i are associated with improved renal outcomes, including reduction in albuminuria, CKD progression, and renal death, a modest decline in eGFR on initiation should not warrant discontinuation of SGLT2i therapy. There is strong evidence from clinical trials that SGLT2i therapy has beneficial cardiovascular and renal effects. Three large RCT's—EMPA-REG, CANVAS, and DECLARE TIMI—all reported a reduction in primary cardiovascular outcomes and secondary renal outcomes. In addition, the CREDENCE trial was specifically designed to investigate renal outcomes, with the primary outcome being a composite of ESRD, that is, dialysis, transplantation, or sustained estimated eGFR of <15 mL/min/1.73 m^2, a doubling of serum creatinine, or death from renal or cardiovascular causes. The canagliflozin group demonstrated a 34% relative risk reduction in the renal-specific composite of ESRD (HR 0.66), and a 32% reduction in RR of ESRD (HR 0.68). Two further RCTs—DAPA-HF and EMPEROR-Reduced—showed a significant reduction in the primary outcome of heart failure or cardiovascular death among patients with reduced ejection fraction, stratified by the presence of type 2 diabetes and an eGFR of <60 and ≥60 mL/min/1.73 m^2.

Further weight is added by the recently published DAPA-CKD, which investigated the effect of dapagliflozin on a composite primary outcome of sustained decline in eGFR of at least 50%, ESRD, or death from renal or cardiovascular causes in CKD patients with an eGFR ranging from 25 to 75 mL/min/1.73 m^2 and severely increased albuminuria (200–5000 mg/g or 20–500 mg/mmol) with and without type 2 diabetes (see table 6.2). There was a 40% RR reduction in the primary outcome in the group receiving dapagliflozin (HR 0.61) and the trial was stopped early due to efficacy.

SGLT2 inhibitors decrease blood glucose levels by inhibiting tubular reabsorption of glucose, resulting in a modest reduction in HbA1c (0.7%) in a large meta-analysis by Vasilakou *et al*. They also produce osmotic diuresis and lowering of systolic BP (4.5 mmHg in the same meta-analysis). However, the cardio- and renoprotective effects appear out of proportion to these

Table 6.2 Cardiovascular and kidney outcome trials for SGLT2 inhibitors

	EMPA-REG	CANVAS	DECLARE-TIMI	CREDENCE	DAPA-CKD
Drug	Empagliflozin 10 mg, 25 mg once daily	Canagliflozin 100 mg, 300 mg once daily	Dapagliflozin 10 mg once daily	Canagliflozin 100 mg once daily	Dapagliflozin 10 mg once daily
Total number of participants	7020	10,142	17,160	4401	4304
N (%) with CVD	7020 (100%)	6656 (66%)	6974 (41%)	2220 (50%)	1610 (37%)
eGFR criteria for enrolment	≥30 mL/min/1.73 m^2	≥30 mL/min/1.73 m^2	CrCl ≥60 mL/min, 45% had eGFR 60–90	30–90 mL/min/1.73 m^2, ACR 300–5000 mg/g	25–75 mL/min/1.73 m^2, ACR 200–5000 mg/g
Mean eGFR at enrolment (mL/min/1.73 m^2)	74	76	85	56	43
N (%) with eGFR <60	1819 (26%)	2039 (20%)	1265 (7.4%)	2592 (59%)	3850 (89%)
ACR	No criteria ACR <30 mg/g (3 mg/mmol) in 60%; 30–300 mg/g (3–30 mg/mmol) in 30%; >300 mg/g (30 mg/mmol) in 10%	No criteria Median ACR 12.3 mg/g (1.23 mg/mmol)	No criteria	Criteria: ACR >300–5000 mg/g (30–500 mg/mmol); median ACR 927 mg/g (92.7 mg/mmol)	Criteria: ACR 200–5000 mg/g (20–500 mg/mmol); median ACR 949 mg/g (94.9 mg/mmol)
Follow-up (median, year)	3.1	2.4	4.2	2.6	2.4
Primary outcome(s)	MACE	MACE	(1) MACE; (2) Composite CV death or hospitalization for HF	Composite kidney	Composite kidney

CV outcome results	MACE: HR 0.86, 95% CI 0.74–0.99 Hospitalization for HF: HR 0.65, 95% CI 0.50–0.85	MACE: HR 0.86, 95% CI 0.75–0.97 Hospitalization for HF: HR 0.67, 95% CI 0.52–0.87	MACE: HR 0.93, 95% CI 0.84–1.03 CV death or hospitalization for HF: HR 0.83, 95% CI 0.73–0.95	CV death, MI, stroke: HR 0.80, 95% CI 0.67–0.95 Hospitalization for HF: HR 0.61, 95% CI 0.47–0.80	CV death: HR 0.81, 95% CI 0.58–1.12 CV death or hospitalization for HF: HR 0.71, 95% CI 0.55–0.92
Kidney outcome	Incident or worsening nephropathy (progression to severely increased albuminuria, doubling of SCr, initiation of KRT, or renal death) and incident albuminuria	Composite doubling in SCr, ESRD, or death from renal causes	Composite of $\geq$40% decrease in eGFR to <60 mL/min/1.73 m^2, ESKD, CV or renal death	Composite of ESRD outcomes, doubling SCr, or death from renal or CV causes	Composite of sustained decline in eGFR of at least 50%, ESRD, or death from renal or CV causes
Kidney outcome results	Incident/worsening nephropathy: 12.7% vs 18.8% in empagliflozin vs placebo (HR 0.61; 95% CI: 0.53–0.70) Incident albuminuria: NS	Composite kidney: 1.5 vs 2.8 1000 patient-years in canagliflozin vs placebo (HR 0.53, 95% CI 0.33–0.84)	Composite kidney: HR 0.76, 95% CI 0.67–0.87	Primary kidney: HR 0.70, 95% CI 0.59–0.82	Primary kidney: HR 0.61, 95% CI 0.51–0.72

Abbreviations: ACR, albumin:creatinine ratio; CI, confidence interval; CrCl, creatinine clearance; CV, cardiovascular; CVD, cardiovascular disease; eGFR, estimated glomerular filtration rate; ESRD, end-stage renal disease; GFR, glomerular filtration rate; HF, heart failure; HR, hazard ratio; KRT, kidney replacement therapy; MACE, major adverse cardiovascular events; MI, myocardial infarction; NS, not significant; SCr, serum creatinine; SGLT2, sodium–glucose cotransporter-2; T2D, type 2 diabetes.

Reproduced with permission from KDIGO 2020 Clinical Practice Guideline for Diabetes Management in Chronic Kidney Disease. *Kidney International*, Vol 98. Issue 4S. 2020.

relatively modest reductions. As such, it is thought that improvements in cardiovascular and renal outcomes are independent of blood glucose lowering and may be brought about by mechanisms such as reduced intra-glomerular pressure, resulting in preservation of renal function. Metformin and SGLT2i both reduce the risk of developing complications of type 2 diabetes and carry a low risk of hypoglycaemia. Metformin is a safe and effective treatment that has demonstrated long-term benefits in reducing diabetes complications. By comparison, SGLT2 inhibitors have a lesser effect on glycaemic control, but large effects on lowering cardiovascular risk and progression of CKD, which appear to be independent of the eGFR. Indeed, a large proportion of patients recruited into the cardiovascular outcome trials of SGLT2i were also on metformin. Furthermore, many patients will require more than one anti-hyperglycaemic agent to achieve glycaemic control. There are little data available comparing the use of metformin vs an SGLT2i in 'drug-naïve' patients, and the suggested approach by KDIGO is to initiate metformin first, with a view to adding in an SGLT2i, where possible, for the added beneficial effects on cardiovascular disease and CKD progression.

KDIGO suggests that once a patient has been commenced on an SGLT2i, it is reasonable to continue treatment, even if the eGFR falls below $30 \, \text{mL/min/1.73 m}^2$, unless the drug is not tolerated or dialysis treatment is initiated. However, a switch should be made to an SGLT2i appropriate to the eGFR; for example, empagliflozin could be replaced with canagliflozin when there is a sustained fall in eGFR to $<40 \, \text{mL/min/1.73 m}^2$. Of note, in the DAPA-CKD trial, dapagliflozin was prescribed for patients with an eGFR of $25 \, \text{mL/min/1.73 m}^2$ with an acceptable safety profile, thus supporting the use of this agent at lower levels of renal function. A further RCT, EMPA-KIDNEY, investigating the effects of empagliflozin 10 mg once a day, compared with placebo, on CKD progression or cardiovascular death in patients with an eGFR of $20 \, \text{mL/min/1.73 m}^2$ showed reduced progression of kidney disease and lower risk of cardiovascular disease in patients with CKD. Patients with type 2 diabetes on SGLT2i have an increased risk of developing euglycaemic diabetic ketoacidosis. Therefore, during periods of prolonged fasting, for example, surgery or procedures or acute severe illness, SGLT2i should be withheld.

The EMPA-KIDNEY Collaborative Group. Design, recruitment, and baseline characteristics of the EMPA-KIDNEY trial. Nephrol Dial Transplant. 2022;37(7):1317–29.

115. B. Dapagliflozin 10 mg once a day.

Up until recently, the United States FDA stipulated that dapagliflozin should not be initiated at eGFR $<45 \, \text{mL/min/1.73 m}^2$. However, as mentioned in the previous question, the DAPA-CKD trial utilized dapagliflozin 10 mg once a day down to an eGFR of $25 \, \text{mL/min/1.73 m}^2$ with no reported adverse effects, thereby supporting the use of this SGLT2i in the patient outlined in this case. In light of these trial data, licensing has now changed, although there is some variation among countries. In the UK, dapagliflozin can now be initiated above an eGFR of $15 \, \text{mL/min/}$ $1.73 \, \text{m}^2$, and in the USA above an eGFR of $25 \, \text{mL/min/1.73 m}^2$ (see table 6.3). Canagliflozin is licensed for initiation in patients with an eGFR $>30 \, \text{mL/min/1.73 m}^2$. The starting dose of canagliflozin is 100 mg once a day and should be taken in the morning before breakfast. The dose can be titrated up to 300 mg once a day in patients with an eGFR of $>60 \, \text{mL/min/1.73 m}^2$. In patients with an eGFR of $30–59 \, \text{mL/min/1.73 m}^2$, the maximum dose is 100 mg once per day. Most recently, the results of EMPA-KIDNEY, published in January 2023, demonstrated a reduction in CKD progression and cardiovascular death in the empagliflozin arm compared with placebo (HR 0.72; 95% CI 0.64 to 0.82; P<0.001). Subjects were included down to an eGFR of $20 \, \text{mL/min/1.73 m}^2$, with just over a third of those included having an eGFR $<30 \, \text{mL/min/1.73 m}^2$. The dose of empagliflozin used in the trial was 10 mgs once a day. The FDA accepted a supplemental New Drug Application in January 2023 following publication of EMPA-KIDNEY. Licensing and incorporation into guidelines are expected to follow

Table 6.3 SGLT2 inhibitor with established kidney and cardiovascular benefits and dose adjustments as approved by the US FDA (take note of country-to-country variation)

SGLT2 inhibitor	Dose	Kidney function eligible for inclusion in pivotal randomized trials	Dosing approved by the US FDA
Canagliflozin	100–300 mg once daily	CANVAS: eGFR ≥30 mL/min/1.73 m² CREDENCE: eGFR 30–90 mL/min/1.73 m²	No dose adjustment if eGFR >60 mL/min/1.73 m² 100 mg daily if eGFR 30–59 mL/min/1.73 m² Avoid initiation with eGFR <30 mL/min/1.73 m², discontinue when initiating dialysis
Dapagliflozin	5–10 mg once daily	DECLARE-TIMI 58: CrCl ≥60 ml/min DAPA-HF: eGFR ≥30 ml/min/1.73 m² DAPA-CKD: eGFR 25–75 mL/min/1.73 m²	No dose adjustment if eGFR ≥45 ml/min/1.73 m² Not recommended with eGFR <25 mL/min/1.73 m² NB. This differs from UK licensing where dapagliflozin can be initiated with eGFR ≥15 ml/min/1.73 m²
Empagliflozin	10–25 mg once daily	EMPA-REG: eGFR ≥30 ml/min/1.73 m² EMPA-KIDNEY: eGFR 20–90 mL/min/1.73 m² EMPEROR-Reduced: eGFR ≥20 ml/min/1.73 m²	No dose adjustment if eGFR ≥45 ml/min/1.73 m² Avoid use, discontinue with eGFR persistently <45 mL/min/1.73 m²

Abbreviations: eGFR, estimated glomerular filtration rate; FDA, Food and Drug Administration; SGLT2i, sodium–glucose cotransporter-2 inhibitor

*N.B. EMPA-KIDNEY, published in January 2023, showed no major difference in serious adverse events between groups. A supplemental NDA has been submitted to the FDA; updates to licensing and guidelines are awaited..

Reproduced with permission from KDIGO 2020 Clinical Practice Guideline for Diabetes Management in Chronic Kidney Disease. *Kidney International*, Vol 98. Issue 45. 2020.

.

National Institute for Health and Care Excellence (2015, updated 2022). Type 2 diabetes in adults: management. NICE guideline [NG28]. Available from: https://www.nice.org.uk/guidance/ng28

116. C. Inhibits active reverse co-transport of sodium and glucose on the luminal surface of the S1 segment of the proximal renal tubule.

Answers : In this question, options describe the mechanism of action of different drugs which are as follows:

a) thiazolidinediones, b) sulphonylureas, d) dipeptidyl-peptidase IV (DPP-4) inhibitors e) glucagon-like-peptide-1 (GLP-1) receptor agonists

Rehani PR, Iftikhar H, Nakajima M, Tanaka T, Jabbar Z, Rehani RN. Safety and mode of action of diabetes medications in comparison with 5-aminolevulinic acid (5-ALA). J Diabetes Res. 2019;2019:4267357.

117. D. Stop losartan.

In general, a rise in serum creatinine (SCr) level after initiation or dose increase of an ACEi or ARB should not deter continuation of therapy, provided the SCr level does not rise by >30% within 4 weeks. Interestingly, in clinical trials, participants with the lowest eGFRs at the start of the study and those who demonstrated an increase in SCr level of up to 30% from baseline that stabilized within 2 months of initiation were conferred the greatest benefit in slowing of CKD progression. As such, small increases in SCr level are to be expected and may simply indicate that the treatment is having the desired effect of reducing the intra-glomerular pressure. However, in patients where the SCr level rises above the threshold of 30%, ACEi or ARB therapy should be suspended, and underlying causative factors explored. Commonly, an acute SCr rise in the setting of ACEi or ARB initiation may be attributed to a reduction in effective circulating blood volume, for example, in volume depletion, heart failure, diuretic, or NSAID use. In addition, and in the case example here patients with atherosclerotic cardiovascular disease may have underlying renal artery stenosis and appropriate investigative imaging should be considered if no other clear cause can be demonstrated for a rise in SCr. The aim should be to restart ACEi or ARB therapy once the underlying cause has been ascertained and managed.

Fu EL, Evans M, Clase CM, Tomlinson LA, et al. Stopping renin-angiotensin system inhibitors in patients with advanced CKD and risk of adverse outcomes: A nationwide study. J Am Soc Nephrol. 2021 Feb;32(2):424–35.

118. B. Start sodium zirconium cyclosilicate.

While all the options are feasible, answer B is most appropriate for the following reasons:

- Emphasis should be placed on continuing ACEi or ARB therapy in a diabetic, hypertensive patient with progressive proteinuric CKD, where possible, due to the established cardiovascular and renal benefits, and every effort should be made to adopt other measures of controlling potassium level before decreasing the dose or stopping the medication altogether.

- Dietary potassium intake should be restricted and counselling by a dietician is appropriate in this setting. However, it is unlikely to correct this patient's hyperkalaemia as a standalone intervention, since some patients find it difficult to comply with a low-potassium diet and other contributory factors, such as secondary hypoaldosteronism, may also be a feature in patients with diabetic nephropathy.

- Treatment with oral sodium bicarbonate is effective in reducing serum potassium levels in patients with CKD and metabolic acidosis. However, this patient's serum bicarbonate is almost corrected to within the normal range and he is already on a relatively high dose of serum bicarbonate, such that increasing the dose further is unlikely to impact upon the potassium level.

- Loop diuretics, such as furosemide, enhance renal potassium excretion and are most useful where there is concurrent fluid overload or hypertension in the setting of hyperkalaemia.

- This patient has moderate hyperkalaemia despite being treated with adequate doses of sodium bicarbonate and there are compelling reasons for angiotensin receptor blockade to continue and for the dose to be increased if tolerated. Dietary potassium restriction is warranted but will not correct the problem of hyperkalaemia alone. The best treatment option is to start a gastrointestinal cation exchanger such as patiromer or sodium zirconium cyclosilicate, both of which are recommended by NICE. Both agents have been shown to be effective in achieving normokalaemia and allowing continuation of ACEi or ARB therapy. Safety data from clinical trials exist for up to 1 year but beyond this are currently unavailable, and cost and accessibility to such treatments in some countries remain a significant barrier.

National Institute for Health and Care Excellence (2020). Patiromer for treating hyperkalaemia. Technology appraisal guidance [TA623]. Available from: https://www.nice.org.uk/guidance/ta623/chapter/1-Recommendations

National Institute for Health and Care Excellence (2020). Sodium zirconium cyclosilicate for treating hyperkalaemia. Technology appraisal guidance [TA599]. Available from: https://www.nice.org.uk/guidance/TA599

119. C. In a meta-analysis, GLP-1 RA resulted in a 17% reduction in a composite kidney outcome, mainly due to a reduction in urine albumin excretion.

Kristensen *et al.* conducted a meta-analysis of seven RCTs of GLP-1 RA: ELIXA (Evaluation of LIXisenatide in Acute Coronary Syndrome), LEADER (Liraglutide Effect and Action in Diabetes: Evaluation of Cardiovascular Outcome Results), SUSTAIN-6 (Trial to Evaluate Cardiovascular and Other Long-term Outcomes with Semaglutide in Subjects with Type 2 Diabetes), EXSCEL (EXenatide Study of Cardiovascular Event Lowering), HARMONY (Effect of Albiglutide, When Added to Standard Blood Glucose Lowering Therapies, on Major Cardiovascular Events in Subjects With Type 2 Diabetes Mellitus), REWIND (Researching Cardiovascular Events With a Weekly Incretin in Diabetes), and PIONEER 6 (Peptide Innovation for Early Diabetes Treatment), comprising a total of 56,004 participants. The authors evaluated pooled cardiovascular and kidney outcome data in the general diabetes population, including patients with CKD. In this meta-analysis, GLP-1 RA was shown to reduce the relative risk for a broad composite kidney outcome (HR 0.83; 95% CI 0.78–0.89; P <0.001) in the general diabetes population, including patients with CKD. In these study groups selected for cardiovascular risk, kidney endpoints were driven largely by reduction in albuminuria. Excluding severely increased albuminuria, the association of GLP-1 RA with kidney endpoints was not significant. A significant limitation of these results is that data have not been reported from study populations selected for CKD or with a kidney-specific primary outcome. To fill this gap, the FLOW (Effect of Semaglutide Versus Placebo on the Progression of Renal Impairment in Subjects With Type 2 Diabetes and Chronic Kidney Disease) trial is currently under way, with the aim of investigating whether semaglutide improves kidney outcomes among participants with type 2 diabetes and CKD (eGFR 25–50 mL/min/1.73 m^2 or with severely increased albuminuria) on a background of standard of care. A further recent trial, Effect of Efpeglenatide on Cardiovascular Outcomes (AMPLITUDE-O), demonstrated a relative risk reduction in a composite kidney endpoint in patients with T2DM and either a history of cardiovascular disease or current CKD (eGFR 25.0–59.9 mL/min/1.73 m^2), with at least one other cardiovascular risk factor, by 32%, adding further weight to the current evidence of benefit from GLP-1 RA on renal outcomes.

Answer A is incorrect. The incretin effect is, in fact, reduced or completely absent in patients with T2DM. GLP-1 is an incretin hormone, which is secreted from the intestine in response to a glucose load and stimulates insulin secretion from the pancreatic islet β-cells. It also enhances weight loss by way of delayed gastric emptying and reduced appetite stimulation in the brain. Answer D is incorrect. In the same meta-analysis as above, Kristensen *et al.* showed that compared with placebo, the GLP-1 RA treatment group had a reduction in cardiovascular death, fatal and non-fatal myocardial infarction, all-cause mortality, and hospitalization for heart failure. This is the first time a benefit in terms of heart failure hospitalization has been demonstrated for the GLP-1 RA class; however, the reduction was not as large as that demonstrated with SGLT2i therapy.

Answer B is incorrect. KDIGO recommends that metformin and an SGLT2i should be used as initial therapy to achieve an individualized HbA1c ranging between <6.5% and <8.0% in patients with T2DM and CKD. A long-acting GLP-1 RA should be used as additional treatment where the glycaemic target has not been achieved or where these medications are not tolerated.

Answer E is incorrect. The risk of hypoglycaemia is low when a GLP-1 RA is used alone. However, when used concomitantly with agents such as insulin or sulfonylureas, the risk of hypoglycaemia is increased. Dose reduction or stopping either insulin or a sulfonylurea should be considered when starting a GLP-1 RA, if it is deemed to be a significant risk of hypoglycaemia.

Gerstein HC, Sattar N, Rosentock J, et al.; AMPLITUDE-O Trial Investigators. Cardiovascular and renal outcomes with efpeglenatide in type 2 diabetes. N Engl J Med. 2021;385:896–907.

Kristensen SL, Rorth R, Jhund PS, *et al*. Cardiovascular, mortality, and kidney outcomes with GLP-1 receptor agonists in patients with type 2 diabetes: a systematic review and meta-analysis of cardiovascular outcome trials. Lancet Diabetes Endocrinol. 2019;7(10):776–85.

120. E. Start liraglutide, stop sitagliptin, and reduce gliclazide.

This patient has progressive CKD with nephrotic-range proteinuria and is at high cardiovascular risk. He is also obese and has not managed to lose weight despite being on metformin and SGLT2i, as well as with added dietary intervention. Of the options, the most appropriate treatment is to commence a GLP-1 RA. KDIGO guidelines stipulate that the choice of GLP-1 RA should prioritize those agents with RCT evidence of cardiovascular benefit, that is, liraglutide, semaglutide (injectable form), and dulaglutide. Importantly, these three agents also showed evidence of improved renal outcomes. Metformin is an effective anti-glycaemic, with a low risk of hypoglycaemia, and KDIGO recommends treating patients with T2DM, CKD, and an eGFR ≥30 mL/min1.73 m^2 with this agent. In patients with an eGFR of 30–45 mL/min/ 1.73 m^2, the maximum dose should be halved. Metformin is not metabolized and is excreted unaltered in the urine. A biguanide called phenformin was withdrawn from the market in 1977 due to an association with lactic acidosis. As a result, the FDA issued a warning against the use of metformin in CKD where drug excretion may be impaired, thereby increasing the risk of lactic acid accumulation. However, evidence for an association between metformin and lactic acidosis has been inconsistent (and, in some cases, even refuted), leading the FDA to change its advice to including patients with an eGFR ≥30 mL/min/1.73 m^2. Below this level of renal function, the agent should be discontinued. Concurrent use of a GLP-1 RA and sulfonylurea may increase the risk of hypoglycaemia. As such, reducing the dose of gliclazide by 50% and advising the patient to monitor his capillary blood glucose at home is appropriate. Stopping gliclazide in this patient is probably unnecessary, given his elevated HbA1c and home capillary blood glucose readings suggesting he is at low risk of hypoglycaemic episodes. GLP-1 RAs should not be used in conjunction with DPP-4 inhibitors. In addition, since GLP-1 RAs offer cardiovascular and renal benefits, stopping sitagliptin in order to facilitate treatment with liraglutide is the best treatment option in this patient. Initiation of insulin degludec is not the correct treatment step, since liraglutide confers cardiovascular risk reduction (a priority in this patient), in addition to lowering HbA1c and targeting weight loss. It is also not appropriate at this stage to commence combination treatment with insulin degludec and liraglutide (before trying liraglutide alone), owing to the risk of hypoglycaemia, especially in the context of concomitant treatment with gliclazide.

Kidney Disease: Improving Global Outcomes Diabetes Work Group. KDIGO 2020 Clinical Practice Guideline for Diabetes Management in Chronic Kidney Disease. Kidney Int Suppl. 2020;98(4S):S1–115.

National Institute for Health and Care Excellence (2020). Type 2 diabetes in adults: management. Published date: February 2022. Last updated: August 2022. https://www.nice.org.uk/guidance/ng28

Take-Home Messages

1. Care of the DKD patient is complex and multifaceted, and a variety of treatment approaches should be used, including lifestyle and dietary interventions and pharmacological treatments for hyperglycaemia, hypertension, and hyperlipidaemia.

2. In general, patients with DKD should be assigned an individualized HbA1c target, based on the need to prevent micro- and macrovascular complications vs the risk of hypoglycaemia and other comorbidities, including severity of CKD and life expectancy.

3. A tighter systolic BP target of <120 mmHg is now recommended by KDIGO for adults with hypertension and CKD; separate targets for albuminuria have now been removed. However,

in the diabetic population, there is no solid evidence that lowering systolic BP to <120 mmHg confers any benefit. In patients with diabetes, KDIGO recommends starting an ACEi or ARB in the presence of hypertension, CKD, and moderately to severely increased albuminuria.

4. There is now a large body of evidence confirming that SGLT-2 inhibitors confer significant reno- and cardioprotective effects in patients with T2DM and CKD. KDIGO recommends treating patients with T2DM, CKD, and an eGFR ≥30 mL/min /1.73 m² with an SGLT-2i. A modest, reversible decrease in eGFR may be observed on initiation of treatment.

5. Once a patient has been commenced on an SGLT2i, it is reasonable to continue treatment, even if the eGFR falls below 30 mL/min/1.73 m², unless the drug is not tolerated or dialysis treatment is initiated. A switch may need to be made according to the eGFR, for example, from empagliflozin to canagliflozin based on current drug licensing.

6. GLP-1 RA have multiple beneficial effects, including improved glycaemic control, weight loss, and reduction in BP. Several of these agents have also demonstrated a reduction in cardiovascular risk, as well as favourable renal outcomes, including reduction in albuminuria and preservation of eGFR. KDIGO recommends a long-acting GLP-1 RA in patients with T2DM and CKD who have not achieved individualized glycaemic targets despite use of metformin and SGLT-2I treatment (or who are unable to use these medications).

7. Finerenone, a selective non-steroidal mineralocorticoid antagonist, has recently been shown to improve both renal and cardiovascular outcomes in people with diabetic kidney disease. As such, it is likely to be included in clinical practice guidelines in the future. Indeed, note is made of the latest draft version of the KDIGO CKD guideline, released in July 2023, which incorporates a recommendation for the use of non-steroidal MRAs in patients with an eGFR ≥25 mL/min/1.73m², normokalaemia and a uACR >3 mg/mmol despite maximum RAS blockade.

chapter 7

CARDIOVASCULAR DISEASE, HYPERTENSION, AND DIABETES (PART B)

QUESTIONS

121. A 63-year-old man was seen in the nephrology clinic with chronic kidney disease secondary to membranous glomerulonephritis. He had no significant past history and was on no regular medications.

On examination, his BP was 164/97 mmHg. He had moderate pitting oedema up to his mid shins bilaterally.

Urinalysis showed protein 1+, blood nil.

Investigations:

serum sodium	140 mmol/L (137–144)
serum potassium	4.6 mmol/L (3.5–4.9)
serum creatinine	147 µmol/L (60–110)
eGFR	42 mL/min/1.73 m^2 (>60)
serum albumin	32 g/L (37–49)
urine albumin:creatinine ratio	24 mg/mmol (<2.5)

What is the most appropriate next step in management?

A. ambulatory BP monitoring
B. amlodipine
C. furosemide
D. prednisolone
E. ramipril

Best of Five MCQs for the European Specialty Examination in Nephrology. Shafi Malik, Oxford University Press.
© Oxford University Press 2024. DOI: 10.1093/oso/9780192844163.003.0013

122. **A 54-year-old man was seen in the nephrology clinic with difficult-to-control BP, tiredness, and daytime somnolence. He suffers from angina and has a previous history of transient ischaemic attack 2 years ago. He was taking amlodipine 10 mg, ramipril 10 mg, indapamide 2.5 mg, and simvastatin 40 mg once daily.**

On examination, his BP was 175/101 mmHg. He had no ankle swelling, and his BMI was 36 kg/m^2.

Urinalysis showed trace protein only.

A 24-hour ambulatory BP monitor showed the following:

daytime BP average	155/95 mmHg
night-time average	158/98 mmHg

Investigations:

serum sodium	137 mmol/L (137–144)
serum potassium	4.9 mmol/L (3.5–4.9)
serum creatinine	123 µmol/L (60–110)
eGFR	53 mL/min/1.73 m^2 (>60)
urine albumin:creatinine ratio	13 mg/mmol (<2.5)

What is the most appropriate next step in management?

A. add bisoprolol

B. add spironolactone

C. assess adherence

D. investigate for secondary causes of hypertension

E. refer for sleep studies

123. **A nephrology consult is sought on a 45-year-old woman who presented with chest pain radiating down her left arm. Her past history includes long-standing history of hypertension. She had no prior history of angina. She is a lifelong non-smoker, lives an active lifestyle, and drinks between 4 and 6 units of alcohol per week. She is taking amlodipine 10 mg and ramipril 10 mg once daily.**

On examination, her BP was 162/94 mmHg and her BMI was 23 kg/m². A bruit could be heard over the abdomen, and the rest of her examination was normal. An ECG showed ST elevation in leads V2 and V3. An echocardiogram showed an ejection fraction of 60%, with left ventricular hypertrophy and no regional wall motion abnormalities.

Investigations:

eGFR	51 mL/min/1.73 m² (>60)
serum cholesterol	3.8 mmol/L (<5.2)
serum HDL-cholesterol	1.5 mmol/L (>1.55)
serum non-HDL-cholesterol	1.3 mmol/L (<3.36)
serum troponin I (baseline)	156 ng/L (<10)
serum troponin I (3 hours)	697 ng/L (<10)

An angiogram of coronary arteries showed a longitudinal filling defect in the left anterior descending artery and there were no atherosclerotic lesions in other coronary segments. A renal angiogram carried out at the same time showed a 'string of beads' appearance of the right renal artery.

What is the most likely underlying diagnosis?

A. acute coronary syndrome

B. fibromuscular dysplasia

C. renal artery dissection

D. renal artery stenosis

E. spontaneous coronary artery dissection

124. **A 77-year-old man presented to the emergency department for the second time in 6 months with progressive breathlessness over 24 hours without any chest pain. He is an ex-smoker of 40 pack-years and has a long-standing history of hypertension and CKD. He was taking amlodipine 10 mg, losartan 50 mg, and indapamide 2.5 mg.**

On examination, chest auscultation revealed fine end-inspiratory crepitations and mild ankle oedema bilaterally. His BP was 173/84 mmHg, heart rate 92 beats/min, respiratory rate 26 breaths/min, and oxygen saturation 92% on room air. An echocardiogram showed an ejection fraction of 55%.

Investigations:

serum sodium	139 mmol/L (137–144)
serum potassium	4.5 mmol/L (3.5–4.9)
serum creatinine	145 µmol/L (60–110)
eGFR	41 mL/min/1.73 m² (>60)
chest X-ray	pulmonary oedema
transthoracic echocardiogram EF	55%

What is the most appropriate next step in management?

A. CT angiography

B. increase the dose of losartan

C. MR angiography

D. renal arterial angiography

E. ultrasound Doppler scan of kidneys

125. **A 67-year-old woman is seen in the nephrology clinic with CKD and hypertension. Her past history includes coronary artery bypass graft surgery 8 years ago and right carotid endarterectomy 5 years ago. She was taking aspirin, amlodipine, bisoprolol, furosemide, doxazosin, and hydralazine. Her adherence was confirmed by a urine antihypertensive screen. She smokes 20 cigarettes per day, with a 40 pack-year history. Her exercise tolerance is limited to 5 minutes of walking due to intermittent claudication in her legs.**

On examination, an abdominal bruit could be heard. Her clinic BP was 156/92 mmHg. A 24-hour ambulatory BP showed the following:

daytime BP average	128/78 mmHg
night-time BP average	137/84 mmHg

Investigations:

serum creatinine	166 µmol/L (60–110)
serum creatinine (6 months ago)	157 µmol/L (60–110)
eGFR	41 mL/min/1.73 m^2 (>60)
plasma renin concentration	high
plasma aldosterone	high

MR angiogram showed 90% ostial stenosis of the right renal artery and 65% stenosis of the left artery.

What is the most appropriate intervention to reduce her cardiovascular risk?

A. right renal artery stenting

B. right renal artery stenting and left renal artery angioplasty

C. right renal sympathetic denervation

D. start ramipril

E. switch bisoprolol and amlodipine to evening time and refer to the smoking cessation clinic

126. **A 37-year-old woman is seen in the nephrology clinic with hypertension. She had no other past history. She was taking ramipril 10 mg, indapamide 2.5 mg, and amlodipine 10 mg. Her adherence was confirmed by a urine antihypertensive screen. She is a lifelong non-smoker, drinks very little alcohol, and leads an active lifestyle. She has a family history of hypertension.**

On examination, her clinic BP was 184/98 mmHg. A 24-hour ambulatory BP showed the following:

daytime BP average	167/95 mmHg
night-time BP average	145/86 mmHg

Investigations:

serum sodium	139 mmol/L (137–144)
serum potassium	3.1 mmol/L (3.5–4.9)
serum cortisol (09.00 h)	normal
plasma metanephrines	normal
plasma renin concentration	undetectable
plasma aldosterone	35 pmol/L (90–720)

The patient was commenced on spironolactone. She returned to the clinic 6 weeks later, following a high-resolution CT scan of the adrenal glands which showed a 17-mm hypodense nodule in the right adrenal. Her repeat clinic BP was 157/89 mmHg.

What is the most appropriate next step in management?

A. adrenal vein sampling
B. fludrocortisone suppression test
C. switch to eplerenone
D. oral sodium loading test
E. right adrenalectomy

127. **A 59-year-old man is seen in the nephrology clinic with stable chronic kidney disease. He had a past history of hypertension. He was taking ramipril 5 mg and amlodipine 10 mg. He is an ex-smoker, drinks very little alcohol, and leads an active lifestyle.**

On examination, his standardized clinic BP was 129/77 mmHg and his BMI was 24.1 kg/m². He had mild ankle oedema bilaterally.

Investigations:

serum sodium	139 mmol/L (137–144)
serum potassium	4.8 mmol/L (3.5–4.9)
serum creatinine	158 µmol/L (60–110)
eGFR	39 mL/min/1.73 m² (>60)
urine albumin:creatinine ratio	57 mg/mmol (<2.5)

What is the most appropriate next step in management?

A. add dapaglifozin and aim for target BP <130/80 mmHg
B. add furosemide and aim for target BP <120/80 mmHg
C. add spironolactone and aim for target BP <120/80 mmHg
D. offer lifestyle advice
E. uptitrate ramipril and aim for target BP <120/80 mmHg

128. **A 20-year-old man is seen in the nephrology clinic after a recent inpatient stay when he presented with headaches and was found to have accelerated hypertension. His BP was initially stabilized with intravenous agents, and he was discharged after his BP was stabilized on amlodipine 10 mg, ramipril 10 mg, and indapamide 2.5 mg.**

   In clinic, he mentioned his father had bleeding in his brain in his thirties and has been on BP-lowering medications since. He had no other past history.

   On examination, his standardized clinic BP was 154/97 mmHg.

   Investigations:
serum creatinine	76 μmol/L (60–110)
serum sodium	142 mmol/L (137–144)
serum potassium	2.9 mmol/L (3.5–4.9)
serum bicarbonate	34 mmol/L (20–28)
plasma renin concentration	low
plasma aldosterone	high

   What is the most appropriate next step in management?

   A. apparent mineralocorticoid excess
   B. excessive liquorice intake
   C. glucocorticoid-remediable aldosteronism
   D. Gordon syndrome
   E. Liddle syndrome

129. **A 51-year-old female lawyer is seen in the nephrology clinic with stable chronic kidney disease and hypertension. She is an ex-smoker with a 10 pack-year history, drinks up to 14 units of alcohol per week, and is a keen marathon runner. She takes ramipril 5 mg daily. On examination, her standardized clinic BP was 122/75 mmHg and her BMI was 22.3 kg/m².**

   Investigations:
   (3 months ago)
eGFR	50 mL/min/1.73 m² (>60)
serum cholesterol	5.4 mmol/L (<5.2)
serum non-HDL-cholesterol	3.4 mmol/L (<3.36)
serum HDL-cholesterol	1.8 mmol/L (>1.55)
fasting serum triglycerides	1.9 mmol/L (0.45–2.30)
urine albumin:creatinine ratio	12 mg/mmol (<2.5)

   She had recently read a news article on cardiovascular disease being the leading cause of morbidity and mortality in patients with chronic kidney disease, and has asked how she can reduce her cardiovascular risk.

   Which of the following interventions would be beneficial in reducing her cardiovascular risk?

   A. dietary modification
   B. increase dose of ramipril
   C. treatment with a statin
   D. treatment with a statin if the estimated 10-year risk of developing CVD is 10% or greater
   E. treatment with ezetimibe

130. **A 75-year-old man presented to the emergency department with progressive exertional breathlessness at rest. His usual exercise tolerance is approximately 250 yards, limited by breathlessness. His past history included chronic kidney disease G4 A3, hypertension, COPD, and congestive cardiac failure.**

    On examination, he was tachypnoeic and unable to complete full sentences. He had fine bibasal inspiratory crepitations and mild peripheral oedema extending up to his knees, and his BP was 145/87 mmHg. His ECG showed 3-mm ST segment depression and T wave inversion in leads II, III, aVF, and V4–V6. His chest X-ray was consistent with changes suggestive of pulmonary oedema. He was started on IV furosemide and an IV infusion of glyceryl trinitrate.

    Investigations:

serum creatinine	245 µmol/L (60–110)
eGFR	22 mL/min/1.73 m^2 (>60)
serum adjusted calcium	2.68 mmol/L (2.20–2.60)
serum phosphate	2.20 mmol/L (0.80–1.45)
serum troponin I (at presentation)	106 ng/L (<10)
serum troponin I (3 hours later)	895 ng/L (<10)

    What is the most appropriate next step in management?

    A. coronary angiography

    B. CT coronary angiography

    C. medical management of acute coronary syndrome

    D. NT-proBNP

    E. transthoracic echocardiography

121. A. Ambulatory BP monitoring.

This patient has stage 1 hypertension based on clinic BP measurement. This, however, needs to be confirmed with either home or ambulatory BP monitoring (NICE guideline). If a patient has diabetes with albuminuria, a urine albumin:creatinine ratio of >70 mg/mmol, or stage 2 hypertension based on clinic BP measurement (BP ≤180/110 mmHg), BP lowering treatment can be started without the need to confirm BP using ambulatory or home monitoring. If clinic BP measurements are obtained in a standardized manner, as suggested in the recent KDIGO guideline on management of BP in CKD, these readings can be used to make decisions on treatment.

In this case, clearly the urine ACR is only mildly raised and therefore would not warrant treatment for membranous nephropathy. As the patient does not have diabetes and only stage 1 hypertension, confirmation of hypertension with ambulatory BP monitoring would be required before starting any antihypertensive treatment. An ambulatory BP monitoring daytime average or home BP monitoring average of 135/85 mmHg or higher would warrant pharmacological treatment.

The recent KDIGO BP guideline suggests that the target systolic BP should be <120 mmHg, when tolerated, using standardized office BP measurement. However, this may not be applicable to all categories of patients with CKD. A more pragmatic BP target for all patients with CKD is <130/80 mmHg, as suggested by the UK Kidney Association.

Dasgupta I, Zoccali C. Is the KDIGO systolic blood pressure target <120 mmHg for chronic kidney disease appropriate in routine clinical practice? Hypertension. 2022;79:4–11.

Kidney Disease: Improving Global Outcomes. KDIGO 2021 Clinical Practice Guideline for the management of blood pressure in chronic kidney disease. Kidney Int. 2021;99:S1–87.

National Institute for Health and Care Excellence (2019). Hypertension in adults: diagnosis and management. NICE guideline [NG136]. Available from: https://www.nice.org.uk/guidance/ng136

National Institute for Health and Care Excellence (2021). Chronic kidney disease: assessment and management. NICE guideline [NG203]. Available from: https://www.nice.org.uk/guidance/ng203

The UK Kidney Association commentary on NICE guideline (NG136). Hypertension in adults: diagnosis and management. Available from: https://ukkidney.org/health-professionals/guidelines/commentary-nice-guideline-ng136-%E2%80%98hypertension-adults-diagnosis-and?msclkid=685522b9b0eb11ec84711ec398b22fbc

122. C. Assess adherence.

This patient has a stage 1 hypertension confirmed on both clinic and ambulatory BP measurements with a white coat effect. He is taking three antihypertensives at maximum doses. He has apparent treatment-resistant hypertension. To confirm true treatment-resistant hypertension, non-adherence to pharmacological treatment should be excluded. Non-adherence may be present in up to half of patients with apparent treatment-resistant hypertension. In patients with treatment resistance, secondary causes of hypertension should also be investigated. Once non-adherence and secondary causes are excluded, both bisoprolol and spironolactone are suitable fourth-line antihypertensives. Although spironolactone has been shown to be superior to both bisoprolol and doxazosin, in this case, bisoprolol is likely to be more beneficial, given the history of angina and a serum potassium level >4.5 mmol/L.

National Institute for Health and Care Excellence (2019). Hypertension in adults: diagnosis and management. NICE guideline [NG136]. Available from: https://www.nice.org.uk/guidance/ng136

123. B. Fibromuscular dysplasia.

This lady does not have any typical risk factors for atherosclerotic coronary artery disease, which is confirmed by the lack of atherosclerotic lesions in the coronary arteries. Instead, the appearance in the LAD described is that of a spontaneous coronary artery dissection.

National Institute for Health and Care Excellence (2019). Hypertension in adults: diagnosis and management. NICE guideline [NG136]. Available from: https://www.nice.org.uk/guidance/ng136

National Institute for Health and Care Excellence (2021). Chronic kidney disease: assessment and management. NICE guideline [NG203]. Available from: https://www.nice.org.uk/guidance/ng203

124. D. Renal arterial angiography.

A combination of unexplained recurrent flash pulmonary oedema with uncontrolled BP points to a diagnosis of renal artery stenosis. In this particular case, it is likely to be of atherosclerotic aetiology. All four imaging modalities can be used to investigate the underlying diagnosis. Reliability of duplex ultrasound is variable and depends on the skill of the ultrasonographer and body habitus of the patient. Both CT and MR angiography are more readily available and are commonly used for screening of renovascular disease. CT angiography requires the use of iodinated contrast, which can increase the risk of contrast nephropathy, especially in patients with pre-existing CKD, and may overestimate the degree of stenosis. MR angiography has the advantage of avoiding exposure to radiation; however, there is a small risk of nephrogenic systemic fibrosis in those with eGFR <30 mL/min. Angiography remains the gold standard for defining the degree of stenosis associated with renovascular disease. The risk of nephrotoxicity remains if an iodinated contrast medium is used, which can be avoided altogether if carbon dioxide is used instead in those with CKD stages 4 and 5. It also allows the operator to deliver a therapeutic intervention in the same sitting if a critical stenosis is identified, and to avoid the need of a separate diagnostic study.

Although RCTs have failed to show that routine renal revascularization has any clinical benefit over best medical therapy, there are three indications for haemodynamically significant renal artery stenosis that would benefit from intervention. These include recurrent 'flash' pulmonary oedema, treatment-resistant hypertension, and progressive renal impairment.

Increasing the dose of losartan is not likely to prevent a future episode of pulmonary oedema. Often the introduction of an ACEi or ARB can unmask the underlying diagnosis by reducing the renal perfusion, leading to a significant reduction in glomerular filtration, especially in the presence of bilateral renal artery stenosis.

Textor SC, Misra S. Does renal artery stenting prevent clinical events? Clin J Am Soc Nephrol. 2016;11(7):1125–7.

125. E. Switch bisoprolol and amlodipine to evening time and refer to the smoking cessation clinic.

This case focusses on management of renal artery stenosis. There is a clear history of widespread atherosclerosis, and the finding of atherosclerotic renal artery disease is not surprising. Indications for renal revascularization have been discussed earlier. In this case, the patient is asymptomatic, BP is well controlled, and renal function is relatively stable. Therefore, the focus of management should be to reduce cardiovascular risk. Patients with CKD often have a reverse dipper pattern on ambulatory blood pressure monitoring which is where night-time BP is elevated and is a stronger prognostic marker of future cardiovascular disease. There is evidence that bedtime administration of antihypertensives may improve cardiovascular risk. Renal sympathetic denervation is a treatment for treatment-resistant hypertension, which is not present here.

Hermida RC, Crespo JJ, Domínguez-Sardiña M, et al. Bedtime hypertension treatment improves cardiovascular risk reduction: the Hygia Chronotherapy Trial. Eur Heart J. 2020;41(48):4565–76.

126. A. Adrenal vein sampling.

This case focusses on secondary causes of hypertension. As per NICE hypertension guidelines, any one with confirmed hypertension who are younger than 40 years or with treatment-resistant hypertension should be investigated for secondary causes of hypertension. Onset of apparent treatment-resistant hypertension at a young age and spontaneous hypokalaemia point to primary hyperaldosteronism. A high serum aldosterone:renin ratio, BP responsive to mineralocorticoid receptor antagonists, and identification of an adrenal nodule all are highly suggestive of primary hyperaldosteronism. The oral sodium loading test and fludrocortisone suppression test are confirmatory tests for primary hyperaldosteronism required in the setting of spontaneous hypokalaemia and plasma renin below detection levels, plus plasma aldosterone concentration (PAC) >20 ng/dL (550 pmol/L). It is worth noting that hypokalaemia may only be present in a minority of patients with primary hyperaldosteronism. Where surgical treatment is desired, adrenal vein sampling (AVS) should be considered to distinguish between unilateral and bilateral adrenal disease, as imaging may not be able to visualize microadenomas. AVS can also distinguish non-functioning incidentalomas from aldosterone-producing adenomas, with confidence, in most patients. Switching to eplerenone will not have any additional benefit.

Funder JW, Carey RM, Mantero F, et al. The management of primary aldosteronism: case detection, diagnosis, and treatment: an Endocrine Society clinical practice guideline. J Clin Endocrinol Metab. 2016;101(5):1889–916.

National Institute for Health and Care Excellence (2019). Hypertension in adults: diagnosis and management. NICE guideline [NG136]. Available from: https://www.nice.org.uk/guidance/ng136

127. E. Uptitrate ramipril and aim for target BP <120/80 mmHg.

The question tests the knowledge of updated KDIGO hypertension guidelines. Significantly, the guidelines have suggested a lower target systolic BP of 120 mmHg, if tolerated. The guidelines have further emphasized the use of standardized clinic BP measurement to improve accuracy and minimize the white coat effect. These changes reflect recent evidence from a subgroup of the SPRINT trial which has suggested the benefit of targeting systolic BP to <120 mmHg, when measured under standardized conditions, by reducing cardiovascular events and all-cause mortality in CKD.

In this case, the patient has moderate albuminuria (>30 mg/mmol) and therefore, RAS inhibition would be the first-line treatment. It should be noted, however, that dual ACE inhibition and angiotensin II receptor blockade is not recommended due to a higher risk of adverse events. In this case, there is room for further optimization of the ramipril dose, given albuminuria, which would be preferable to starting furosemide. The ankle oedema is only mild and likely to be a side effect of amlodipine. Lifestyle advice should be offered in all cases. Salt restriction, Dietary Approaches to Stop Hypertension diet, smoking cessation, and regular exercise have all been shown to improve BP control.

Cheung A, Rahman M, Reboussin D, et al. Effects of intensive BP control in CKD. J Am Soc Nephrol. 2017;28(9): 2812–23.

Kidney Disease: Improving Global Outcomes. KDIGO 2021 Clinical Practice Guideline for the Management of Blood Pressure in Chronic Kidney Disease. Kidney Int. 2021;99:S1–87.

The SPRINT Research Group; Wright JT Jr., Williamson JD, Whelton PK, et al. A randomized trial of intensive versus standard blood-pressure control. N Engl J Med. 2015;373(22):2103–16.

128. C. Glucocorticoid-remediable aldosteronism.

This question tests knowledge of genetic causes of hypertension, which is implied by the family history in a young patient presenting with accelerated hypertension. In addition, the patient has hypokalaemia, metabolic alkalosis, and high serum aldosterone and low serum renin levels. Gordon syndrome is associated with hyperkalaemia and metabolic acidosis.

All other options would cause hypertension-associated hypokalaemia, metabolic alkalosis, and low renin levels. However, only glucocorticoid-remediable aldosteronism is associated with high aldosterone levels, whereas a low aldosterone level is a feature of Liddle syndrome, apparent mineralocorticoid excess, and excessive liquorice intake. Glucocorticoid-remediable aldosteronism is a monogenic form of hypertension with an autosomal dominant inheritance pattern. Abnormal expression of a chimeric gene on chromosome 8 results in biosynthesis of aldosterone in the zona fasciculata of the adrenal gland, which is normally responsible only for cortisol synthesis. Patients often present with typical features of primary hyperaldosteronism with early-onset hypertension, which, if left undiagnosed, poses a high risk of haemorrhagic stroke. Treatment with low-dose corticosteroid is effective, which leads to suppression of blood aldosterone levels.

129. C. Treatment with a statin.

Cardiovascular risk reduction is a key aspect of long-term management in CKD patients. This patient has well-controlled BP, although it is still a bit shy of KDIGO's recommended target systolic BP of <120 mmHg. The patient also has mild albuminuria. Therefore, an argument could be made to increase the dose of ramipril. Her potassium level is already borderline high and any further increases in the dose of ramipril may cause hyperkalaemia. KDIGO recommends starting a statin in any one above the age of 50 years with eGFR <60 mL/min regardless of the cholesterol level or the 10-year cardiovascular risk. KDIGO guidelines do not recommend regular measurements of lipid levels after starting a statin, nor do they suggest a target level of cholesterol. NICE lipid guidelines, by contrast, recommend aiming for a 40% reduction of total cholesterol from baseline level. In the UK, the NICE 2014 lipid guidelines recommend using QRISK2 to estimate the 10-year cardiovascular risk but advised against its use for anyone with eGFR <60 mL/min, as they should be considered to be at an increased risk of cardiovascular disease events without using QRISK2.

Kidney Disease: Improving Global Outcomes. KDIGO Clinical Practice Guideline for lipid management in chronic kidney disease. Kidney Int Suppl. 2013;3:259.

National Institute for Health and Care Excellence (2014). Cardiovascular disease: risk assessment and reduction, including lipid modification. Clinical guideline [CG181]. Available from: https://www.nice.org.uk/guidance/cg181

130. A. Coronary angiography.

Patients with CKD are at high risk of cardiovascular disease and often present in an atypical fashion; breathlessness without chest pain is the typical presenting feature of myocardial ischaemia in this group of patients. This patient has presented with non-ST elevation myocardial infarction (NSTEMI), and evidence suggests myocardial revascularization performed in the shortest period of time in CKD patients, even in the case of NSTEMI, improves prognosis and minimizes the risk of haemodynamic instability. Medical management therefore would be suboptimal therapy in this case. Transthoracic echocardiography may identify regional wall motion abnormalities, which indicate underlying ischaemia, but it does not treat the underlying pathology. CT coronary angiography is used in patients with stable angina. In this case, it is not likely to be useful in a patient with long-standing CKD who has evidence of hyperparathyroidism and therefore may have significant coronary artery calcification which will affect visualization of coronary artery stenosis and may also lead to overestimation of luminal stenosis. NT-proBNP biomarker, alongside severely impaired renal function, may be useful predictors in identifying patients with acute coronary syndrome and CKD who are likely to develop acute pulmonary oedema. In this case, however, the patient has already developed pulmonary oedema and this would not change management.

Take-Home Messages

1. BP measurement in the clinic should be done in a standardized manner by using guidelines from the British and Irish Hypertension Society or KDIGO.
2. Ambulatory or home BP monitoring should be used to confirm the diagnosis of hypertension, especially to rule out the white coat effect and masked hypertension.
3. Spironolactone is the preferred fourth-line treatment option for patients with treatment-resistant hypertension.
4. Adherence testing should be considered in patients with apparent treatment-resistant hypertension.
5. Screening for secondary causes should be performed in patients younger than 40 years with high BP and in those with treatment-resistant hypertension.
6. Revascularization for renal artery stenosis may be considered in selected patients with recurrent flash pulmonary oedema or those with treatment-resistant hypertension.
7. Adrenal vein sampling should be considered to distinguish between unilateral and bilateral adrenal disease.
8. An ACE inhibitor or an angiotensin receptor blocker should be preferentially used in patients with CKD who have hypertension and moderate albuminuria (ACR >30 mg/mmol).

131. **A 20-year-old man is referred for investigation of mild proteinuria. He was otherwise well and has no significant past history.**

Investigations:
serum creatinine   60 µmol/L (60–110)
urine albumin:creatinine ratio   7.5 mg/mmol (<2.5)
ultrasound scan of kidneys   normal-sized kidneys, 4-mm stone in the lower pole of his left kidney

What is the most appropriate management step?

A. open surgery
B. percutaneous nephrolithotomy
C. shock wave lithotripsy
D. ureteroscopy
E. watchful waiting

132. **A 40-year-old man presents with a history of passing a stone per urethra. The stone is sent for analysis and is reported as being a calcium oxalate stone.**

What would you advise the patient?

A. avoid animal protein and reduce dietary calcium
B. avoid spinach and increase dietary calcium
C. daily vitamin C and more animal protein
D. daily vitamin C and more spinach
E. increase intake of nuts and reduce dietary calcium

Best of Five MCQs for the European Specialty Examination in Nephrology. Shafi Malik, Oxford University Press.
© Oxford University Press 2024. DOI: 10.1093/oso/9780192844163.003.0015

133. **A 24-year-old man is seen in the renal outpatient clinic with a history of passing urinary stones. He says he has been passing stones since his teens. He was adopted and was unable to give a family history.**

Investigations:

urine microscopy	hexagonal crystals, and on addition of cyanide nitroprusside, the urine turns purple
ultrasound scan of kidney	normal-sized kidneys, with a staghorn calculus on the right

What would be the most appropriate advice to give?

A. avoid potassium citrate and acetazolamide

B. avoid sodium citrate and sodium bicarbonate

C. increase meat-based protein

D. restrict fluid intake

E. start D-penicillamine

134. **A 40-year-old man is seen in the renal clinic with a 1-week history of right loin pain. He says he may have passed a small stone, though he is not completely certain. He has no significant past history and is not taking any medications.**

What would be the most appropriate investigation?

A. intravenous pyelography

B. MRI with gadolinium

C. non-contrast CT scan

D. plain abdominal X-ray

E. ultrasound scan

135. **A 40-year-old woman presented to emergency department with a history of lower abdominal pain and haematuria. She had no significant past history and was not on any regular medication. While awaiting blood test results, she passed a stone per urethra, which was sent for analysis.**

Urinalysis	struvite stone
Urine pH	6.0 (4.5–8)

What would be the next appropriate step?

A. antibiotics

B. cranberry juice

C. D-penicillamine

D. potassium citrate

E. shock wave lithotripsy

136. A 30-year-old woman is referred to the renal outpatient clinic with a history of passing renal stones. She gives a history of passing a stone a few months ago that was sent for analysis by her GP and was reported as being a calcium oxalate stone.

Investigations:
serum creatinine   74 µmol/L (60–110)
ultrasound scan of kidneys   normal-sized kidneys, no renal calculi seen

What would be the next management step?

A. allopurinol
B. avoid drinking tea
C. drink at least 2 L of water a day
D. sodium bicarbonate with sodium citrate
E. thiazide diuretic and low-sodium diet

137. You are called by a junior doctor about a 36-year-old man who is known to have HIV. He had presented to emergency department 2 days ago with fever, confusion, and a seizure. On admission, he was seen by the infectious diseases team who started him on IV aciclovir and ceftriaxone. The patient is now complaining of abdominal pain.

On examination, his GCS was 15/15.

Investigations:
serum creatinine   360 µmol/L (60–110)
serum creatinine 2 days ago   97 µmol/L (60–110)

What would be the next best step?

A. haemodialysis
B. IV fluids with a loop diuretic
C. morphine
D. start indinavir
E. stop ceftriaxone

138. You are asked to see a 32-year-old woman who is 10 weeks pregnant. She presented to hospital with a 2-day history of acute right-sided abdominal pain associated with fever and haematuria.

On examination, her temperature was 37.9°C and her BP was 110/70 mmHg. She is tender over her left flank.

Investigations:
serum creatinine   110 µmol/L (60–110)
ultrasound scan of kidneys   right-sided hydronephrosis with an 8-mm stone in the renal pelvis, normal left kidney

What is the next appropriate management step?

A. CT scan with contrast
B. IV fluid and observation
C. IV fluid and tamsulosin
D. nephrostomy and antibiotics
E. shock wave therapy

139. **A 56-year-old woman with a history of recurrent urinary tract infections was admitted to hospital with urinary sepsis. She was on trimethoprim prophylaxis. Urine culture grew *Pseudomonas aeruginosa* sensitive to meropenem. The patient was treated with a course of intravenous meropenem and was ready for discharge.**

What would be the next best step for prophylaxis

A. amoxicillin

B. ciprofloxacin

C. fosfomycin

D. no prophylaxis

E. trimethoprim

140. **A 70-year-old person is admitted to hospital with emphysematous pyelonephritis. The patient is known to have hypertension and type 2 diabetes. They were allergic to penicillin.**

On examination, pulse rate was 98 beats/min and his BP was 86/50 mmHg.

Which empirical antibiotic would you prescribe?

A. amoxicillin

B. ciprofloxacin

C. meropenem

D. piperacillin/tazobactam

E. trimethoprim

141. **A 56-year-old person is admitted to hospital with chest pain. They were known to have CKD stage 4, with a baseline serum creatinine level of 180 μmol/L.**

Investigations:	
serum urea	20 mmol/L (2.5–7.0)
serum potassium	5.6 mmol/L (3.5–4.9)
serum creatinine	290 μmol/L (60–110)
ultrasound scan of kidneys	severe bilateral hydroureter and hydronephrosis, with mild cortical thinning

What would be the most appropriate management step?

A. antegrade nephrostomy

B. calcium resonium

C. cystoscopy

D. haemodialysis

E. urinary catheterization

142. **A 43-year-old person manages to pass a renal stone, which is sent for stone analysis and is confirmed as a calcium oxalate stone.**

    Which of the food products should he avoid?

    A. blueberries
    B. broccoli
    C. kale
    D. spinach
    E. sweet potato

143. **A 43-year-old person manages to pass a renal stone, which is sent for stone analysis and is confirmed as a calcium oxalate stone.**

    What would you advise the patient to do?

    A. cranberry juice
    B. drink plenty of water
    C. high-calcium diet
    D. high-protein diet
    E. low-calcium diet

144. **A 24-year-old person presents to hospital with lower back pain. They did not have any significant past history and were not taking any regular medications.**

    Investigations:
    serum urea   4 mmol/L (2.5–7.0)
    serum creatinine   90 µmol/L (60–110)
    ultrasound scan of kidneys   a 5-mm distal ureteric stone in the right ureter

    What would be the next best step?

    A. antegrade nephrostomy
    B. finasteride
    C. lithotripsy
    D. retrograde nephrostomy
    E. tamsulosin

145. **A 54-year-old person presents to hospital with lower back pain. They did not have any significant past history and were not taking any regular medications.**

    Investigations:
    serum urea   15 mmol/L (2.5–7.0)
    serum creatinine   150 µmol/L (60–110)
    ultrasound scan of kidneys   a 3-mm proximal ureteric stone in the right ureter

    What would be the next best step?

    A. finasteride
    B. lithotripsy
    C. nephrostomy
    D. symptomatic treatment
    E. urinary catheterization

131. E. Watchful waiting.

Asymptomatic stones smaller than 5 mm are not likely to affect quality of life and may be passed spontaneously. Watchful waiting for such stones is recommended by NICE. Stones larger than 5 mm may also pass out spontaneously but are more likely to be associated with complications, such as infection, bleeding, or obstruction, and become symptomatic.

National Institute for Health and Care Excellence (2019). Renal and ureteric stones: assessment and management. NICE guideline [NG118]. Available from: https://www.nice.org.uk/guidance/ng118

132. B. Avoid spinach and increase dietary calcium.

Spinach is known to be rich in oxalate. High dietary calcium binds oxalate in the intestines, thus reducing dietary oxalate absorption. Vitamin C, animal protein, and nuts, such as peanuts, almonds, and cashew, are associated with oxalate stones.

Taylor EN, Curhan GC. Diet and fluid prescription in stone disease. Kidney Int. 2006;70:835.

133. B. Avoid sodium citrate and sodium bicarbonate.

Cystine stones account for only about 1–2% of all kidney stones but represent roughly 6–8% of all paediatric calculi. Eighty per cent of cystinuria patients will have their first stone during their first two decades of life. A history of renal stones early in life, large or recurrent kidney stones, and a family history of kidney stones should raise suspicion of cystinuria. The diagnosis can be established by stone analysis, with urine microscopy typically showing pathognomonic hexagonal stones, or by genetic testing. A positive urine cyanide nitroprusside test suggests high cystine levels. Initial treatment consists of increasing fluid intake (aiming for a urine output of >2 L), restriction of sodium, animal protein, and urine alkalinization to a pH of >7 to encourage cystine solubilization. Potassium citrate would help in alkalinization. Although sodium bicarbonate may help in alkalinization, it is associated with a high sodium load and has the adverse effect of promoting cystine excretion. If conservative measures fail, a thiol-containing drug, such as tiopronin or D-penicillamine should be prescribed.

Metabolic Nephropathy Workgroup of the European Reference Network for Rare Kidney Diseases (ERKNet) and eUROGEN. Cystinuria: clinical practice recommendation. Kidney Int. 2021;99(1):48.

134. C. Non-contrast CT scan.

The preferred test for renal stones is a low-dose non-contrast CT scan. Radiolucent stones, such as uric acid stones, are often missed on plain abdominal X-rays. Intravenous pyelography (also called intravenous urography) detects hydronephrosis but is less sensitive and specific than CT scan for detecting renal stones. MRI scan is not useful for detecting stones. It, however, can be used in pregnant women to localize obstruction seen on ultrasound scan. Gadolinium contrast is not usually used and must be avoided in pregnant women. Ultrasound scan is useful for use in pregnant women with suspected renal stones. It is operator-dependent and less accurate than non-contrast CT scan, and small stones can be missed.

Song L, Maalouf NM. Nephrolithiasis. In: KR Feingold, B Anawalt, A Boyce, et al., eds. Endotext. South Dartmouth, MA: MDText.com, Inc., 2000– (updated 2020). Available from: https://www.ncbi.nlm.nih.gov/books/NBK279069/

135. A. Antibiotics.

Struvite is the name given to stones that form in the presence of urease-producing bacteria such as *Proteus mirabilis* and *Klebsiella pneumoniae*, also known as infection stones. The three key principles of treating struvite stones are: removal of all stone fragments, use of antibiotics to treat the infection, and prevention of recurrence. Management includes use of urease inhibitors, acidification therapy, dissolution therapy, extracorporeal shock wave lithotripsy, ureteroscopy, percutaneous nephrolithotomy (PCNL), and anatrophic nephrolithotomy. PCNL is considered to be the gold standard approach to treating struvite calculi. An initial course of antibiotics is appropriate, while working the patient up for possible surgical intervention following imaging. Struvite stones need acidifying urine, where potassium citrate will alkalinize the urine. Cranberry juice may be indicated in recurrent urinary tract infections, although randomized controlled trials have not shown any benefit.

Flannigan R, Choy WH, Chew B, Lange D. Renal struvite stones—pathogenesis, microbiology, and management strategies. Nat Rev Urol. 2014 Jun;11(6):333–41.

Kadlec AO, Fridirici ZC, Acosta-Miranda AM, et al. Bilateral urinary calculi with discordant stone composition. World J Urol. 2014 Feb;32(1):281–5.

136. E. Thiazide diuretic and low-sodium diet.

Low fluid intake will reduce urine output and thus increase the concentration of stone-forming substances such as calcium and oxalate. Patients should be advised to drink sufficient amounts to regularly pass at least 2 L of urine a day.

Xanthine oxidase inhibitors, such as allopurinol, should be reserved for patients who continue to form uric acid stones despite increased fluid intake and urinary alkalinization. Calcium is reabsorbed passively along the concentration gradient created by sodium and water reabsorption in the proximal tubule. A low sodium intake will therefore encourage sodium and calcium reabsorption.

Raising plasma bicarbonate concentration can increase calcium reabsorption and reduce calcium excretion. Citrate loosely binds to calcium in the urine, thus reducing its availability for binding to oxalate or phosphate. However, the extra sodium associated with sodium bicarbonate or sodium citrate will increase sodium and hence calcium excretion, and counter the effect of raising the plasma bicarbonate level.

Thiazide diuretics are thought to reduce urine calcium excretion by causing mild volume depletion, which leads to sodium, and hence calcium, reabsorption. Studies have shown a significant reduction in stone formation, although efficacy is increased if sodium is simultaneously restricted. Tea and coffee were previously thought to be rich in oxalates. However, several studies have shown higher coffee and tea intake were associated with a lower risk of stone formation.

Ferraro PM, Taylor EN, Gambaro G, Curhan GC. Soda and other beverages and the risk of kidney stones. Clin J Am Soc Nephrol. 2013 Aug;8(8):1389–95.

Khan SR, Pearle MS, Robertson WG, Gambaro G, Canales BK, Doizi S, Traxer O, Tiselius HG. Kidney stones. Nat Rev Dis Primers. 2016 Feb 25;2:16008.

137. B. IV fluids with a loop diuretic.

Aciclovir crystals typically form 24–48 hours after starting treatment. They can lead to acute urinary tract obstruction associated with abdominal pain. Treatment generally consists of stopping aciclovir and conservative management with intravenous saline and a loop diuretic to flush out crystals. Urine microscopy may show birefringent needle-shaped crystals under polarized light. Prognosis is good, with recovery usually occurring 4–9 days after stopping aciclovir. Haemodialysis clears aciclovir but does not alter the natural history of the AKI. However, if neurotoxicity occurs in severe aciclovir-associated AKI, haemodialysis may be indicated. Indinavir can cause AKI associated with crystal formation and nephrolithiasis.

Matlaga BR, Shah OD, Assimos DG. Drug-induced urinary calculi. Rev Urol. 2003;5(4):227–31.

Schwartz BF, Schenkman N, Armenakas NA, Stoller ML. Imaging characteristics of indinavir calculi. J Urol. 1999 Apr;161(4):1085–7.

138. D. Nephrostomy and antibiotics.

The preferred imaging modality for suspected stones in pregnant women is an ultrasound scan. Lying the patient on the side with the affected side up may be helpful in distinguishing between hydronephrosis due to an obstructing stone from pregnancy-associated physiological hydronephrosis. If necessary, an MRI scan or low-dose CT scan can be performed. Most stones pass spontaneously because of the physiological dilatation of the urinary tract during pregnancy. Passage can be aided by lying the patient with the affected side up and by use of intravenous fluids. Tamsulosin is not recommended due to limited data on its safety in pregnancy.

Indications for surgical treatment include an obstructing stone with a urinary tract infection or AKI. Given the likelihood of AKI and an obstructed infected system, initial treatment should include a nephrostomy or stent insertion. Stents often get encrusted during pregnancy and require replacing every 4–6 weeks. Obstructing stones may be removed during pregnancy by ureteroscopy and laser lithotripsy, but this should be delayed until the second or third trimester. Shock wave lithotripsy and percutaneous nephrolithotomy for large-volume stones are contraindicated in pregnancy.

Ordon M, Dirk J, Slater J, Kroft J, Dixon S, Welk B. Incidence, treatment, and implications of kidney stones during pregnancy: A matched population-based cohort study. J Endourol. 2020 Feb;34(2):215–21.

Thongprayoon C, Vaughan LE, Chewcharat A, Kattah AG, Enders FT, Kumar R, Lieske JC, Pais VM, Garovic VD, Rule AD. Risk of symptomatic kidney stones during and after pregnancy. Am J Kidney Dis. 2021 Sep;78(3):409–17.

139. D. No prophylaxis.

A prolonged course of antibiotic may help in bladder epithelial healing. However, prophylactic antibiotic use has been associated with development of antimicrobial resistance. There is a 50% risk of patients developing a UTI after stopping prophylactic antibiotics, which also means a significant number of patients may not develop a UTI.

Albert X, Huertas I, Pereiro I, Sanfélix J, Gosalbes V, Perrotta C. Antibiotics for preventing recurrent urinary tract infection in non-pregnant women. Cochrane Database Syst Rev. 2004;3:CD001209.

140. C. Meropenem.

Treatment should target Gram-negative bacteria. In a patient with septic shock, meropenem would be a better choice. The cross-reactivity between meropenem and penicillin is reported to be about 1%, due to structural differences in its side chains and the beta lactam core.

Cunha BA, Hamid NS, Krol V, Eisenstein L. Safety of meropenem in patients reporting penicillin allergy: lack of allergic cross reactions. J Chemother. 2008;20(2):233–7.

Pontin AR, Barnes RD. Current management of emphysematous pyelonephritis. Nat Rev Urol. 2009;6(5):272–9.

141. E. Urinary catheterization.

Causes of hydronephrosis could be split into intrinsic and extrinsic. Intrinsic obstruction may be due to renal calculi, malignancy, ureteropelvic junction stenosis, ureteral strictures, posterior urethral valves, benign prostatic hyperplasia, or neurogenic bladder. Causes of extrinsic compression include pregnancy, malignancy, trauma, and retroperitoneal fibrosis, among others. When there is bilateral hydronephrosis, obstruction distal to the bladder must be suspected, in which case a urinary catheter must be promptly inserted. Cystoscopy-guided stent insertion or an antegrade nephrostomy may be performed as the next step. The patient does not have severe hyperkalaemia, and there is no indication for haemodialysis or calcium resonium.

Thotakura R, Anjum F. Hydronephrosis and hydroureter. In: *StatPearls*. Treasure Island, FL: StatPearls Publishing; 2022. Available from: https://www.ncbi.nlm.nih.gov/books/NBK563217/

142. D. Spinach.

Spinach is high in oxalate. The rest of the food options are low in oxalate.

Trinchieri A. Diet and renal stone formation. Minerva Med. 2013;104(1):41–54.

143. B. Drink plenty of water.

In order to reduce future stone formation, it is essential for patients to drink plenty and be able to pass approximately 2–3 L of urine. None of the other options would be appropriate.

Gul Z, Monga M. Medical and dietary therapy for kidney stone prevention. Korean J Urol. 2014;55(12):775–9.

144. E. Tamsulosin.

Tamsulosin has been shown to be effective in small, distal ureteric stones of 5–10 mm in size, and is now recommended by NICE.

National Institute for Health and Care Excellence (2019). Renal and ureteric stones: assessment and management. NICE guideline [NG118]. https://www.nice.org.uk/guidance/ng118

145. D. Symptomatic treatment.

Symptomatic treatment with an NSAID should be offered first in such cases prior to any intervention. Small stones of 5–10 mm in size are likely to pass on their own.

Leslie SW, Sajjad H, Murphy PB. Renal calculi. In: *StatPearls*. Treasure Island, FL: StatPearls Publishing; 2022. Available from: https://www.ncbi.nlm.nih.gov/books/NBK442014/

Take-Home Messages

1. Asymptomatic stones smaller than 5 mm are not likely to affect quality of life and may be passed spontaneously.
2. High dietary calcium binds oxalate in the intestines, thus reducing dietary oxalate absorption. Vitamin C, animal protein, and nuts, such as peanuts, almonds, and cashew, are associated with oxalate stones.

3. If conservative measures fail, a thiol-containing drug, such as tiopronin or D-penicillamine, is used for treatment of cystine stones.

4. Low-dose non-contrast CT is the imaging modality of choice for renal stones; however, an ultrasound scan may be useful in pregnant women.

5. The key principles of treating struvite stones are: removal of stone fragments, use of antibiotics to treat the infection, and prevention of recurrence. Management includes use of urease inhibitors, acidification therapy, and dissolution therapy.

6. Conservative treatment of stones includes increased fluid intake in order to pass >2 L of urine and alkalinization of the urine (except struvite and calcium phosphate stones where the urine should be acidified).

7. Thiazide diuretics are thought to reduce urine calcium excretion by causing mild volume depletion which leads to sodium, and hence calcium, reabsorption.

8. In cystine stones, urine microscopy typically shows pathognomonic hexagonal stones. A positive urine cyanide nitroprusside test suggests high cystine levels.

146. **A 28-year-old man was seen in the transplant assessment clinic. He is on peritoneal dialysis due to Alport syndrome, with a confirmed mutation in the collagen gene *COL4A5*. His 50-year-old mother is keen to donate a kidney to her son. She has no significant past history and there are no other potential live donors.**

    Which of the following would be an absolute contraindication for his mother to donate?

    A. carrier for *COL4A5* mutation
    B. current smoker
    C. early morning urine ACR 40 mg/mmol
    D. measured GFR 85 mL/min
    E. non-visible haematuria

147. **A 35-year-old woman is referred to the renal clinic with symptomatic hypokalaemia and weight loss over a 12-month period. She denies any gastrointestinal or urinary symptoms.**

    On examination, her BP was 105/60 mmHg, with a postural drop of 15 mmHg. Physical examination was otherwise unremarkable.

    Urinalysis was negative for blood and protein.
    Investigations:
serum creatinine	76 μmol/L (60–110)
serum potassium	2.7 mmol/L (3.5–4.9)
serum bicarbonate	37 mmol/L (20–28)
serum magnesium	0.8 mmol/L (0.75–1.05)
24-h urine potassium	150 mmol (25–120)
24-h urine calcium	6.0 mmol (2.5–7.5)

    Which is the most likely diagnosis?

    A. Bartter syndrome
    B. Gitelman syndrome
    C. proximal renal tubular acidosis
    D. diuretic use
    E. laxative use

Best of Five MCQs for the European Specialty Examination in Nephrology. Shafi Malik, Oxford University Press.
© Oxford University Press 2024. DOI: 10.1093/oso/9780192844163.003.0017

148. **A 56-year-old woman was seen in the transplant clinic. She received a live donor renal transplant from her husband 6 months ago. The HLA mismatch was 1-1-1, with a cold ischaemic time of 3 hours. Her past history included small bowel resection for inflammatory bowel disease. The cause of ESRD was presumed to be interstitial nephritis due to mesalazine. She was currently taking tacrolimus and mycophenolate mofetil.**

Investigations:

serum creatinine (current)   170 µmol/L (60–110)
serum creatinine (baseline)   100 µmol/L (60–110)
blood tacrolimus (trough)   6.0 nmol/L (8.0–12.0)
BK viral load   700 copies/mL (lower detection limit 400)
ultrasound scan of renal transplant   normal perfusion, no hydronephrosis
                                  transplant biopsy (see Fig)

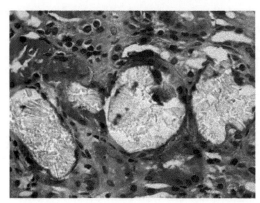

Reproduced with permission from Geraghty, R., Wood, K. & Sayer, J.A. *Urolithiasis* 48, 377–384 (2020). https://doi.org/10.1007/s00240-020-01202-w.

Which is the most appropriate next step in management?

A. amoxicillin

B. calcium carbonate

C. cidofovir

D. infliximab

E. methylprednisolone

149. **An 18-year-old patient is seen in the adult transition clinic. She was diagnosed with nephrotic syndrome aged 14. Her proteinuria did not respond to steroid treatment and she was started on low-dose ciclosporin. Subsequent renal biopsy confirmed focal segmental glomerulosclerosis. She is being worked up for renal transplant. Current medications comprise ciclosporin, ramipril, and furosemide.**

On examination, she was euvolaemic and her BP was 124/80 mmHg.

Investigations:

serum creatinine	220 µmol/L (60–110)
serum albumin	31 g/dL (35–40)
urine albumin:creatinine ratio	430 mmol/L (<2.5)

Genetic screen showed a mutation in the formin gene *INF2*.

What is the most appropriate next step?

A. genetic counselling should be offered as part of conception planning

B. immunosuppression should be continued long term

C. live donation from family members is contraindicated

D. pre-transplant treatment with rituximab

E. stop transplant workup as recurrent disease risk is high

150. **A 52-year-old woman is referred to the renal clinic with malaise, bone pain, and muscle wasting. She has a long past history of dry eyes and mouth. She has used ibuprofen regularly for the last 2 years for joint pain.**

Urinalysis showed protein 1+, blood trace, and glucose negative.

Investigations:

serum sodium	138 mmol/L (137–144)
serum potassium	2.4 mmol/L (3.5–4.9)
serum bicarbonate	10 mmol/L (20–28)
serum phosphate	0.54 mmol/L (0.80–1.45)
serum creatinine	126 µmol/L (60–110)
ultrasound scan of kidneys	bilateral nephrocalcinosis

What is the most likely diagnosis?

A. acquired Fanconi syndrome

B. Gitelman syndrome

C. type 1 renal tubular acidosis

D. type 2 renal tubular acidosis

E. type 4 renal tubular acidosis

151. **A 37-year-old man is referred to the renal clinic after a routine blood test performed by his GP showed abnormal renal function. He is known to have hypertension and gout since his early twenties. He had no siblings but had a family history of renal disease affecting his mother, maternal uncle, and maternal grandfather. Medications included ramipril 5 mg daily, allopurinol 200 mg daily, and diclofenac when required.**

Urinalysis was negative for blood and protein.

Investigations:

serum creatinine	147 µmol/L (60–110)
ultrasound scan of kidneys	normal-sized kidneys, with good corticomedullary definition and no hydronephrosis

Which gene mutation is the most likely explanation for his renal impairment?

A. *COL4A5*
B. *MUC1*
C. *NPHP1*
D. *PKD1*
E. *UMOD*

152. **A 17-year-old man was referred by his GP to the renal outpatient clinic with abnormal renal function. He had recently arrived from Pakistan and was reportedly investigated by an endocrinologist in Pakistan when he was 6 years old for polydipsia and polyuria. He was advised to see a nephrologist but was lost to follow-up.**

On examination, he was pale, and had nystagmus and mild photophobia. He had pitting oedema up to his mid shins. His JVP was +4 cm above the sternal angle, and his BP was 155/80 mmHg.

Investigations:

serum sodium	132 mmol/L (137–144)
serum potassium	5.8 mmol/L (3.5–4.9)
eGFR	14.8 mL/min/1.73 m² (>60)
timed cortisol (09.00 h)	480 nmol/L (320–700)

Ultrasound scan of abdomen: the liver demonstrated a heterogenous echotexture; there was evidence of portal hypertension and mild splenomegaly. Left kidney size 91 mm, right kidney 87 mm in length; both kidneys demonstrated decreased corticomedullary differentiation and occasional small cysts.

Which is the most likely diagnosis?

A. adrenoleukodystrophy
B. autosomal recessive PKD
C. medullary sponge kidney
D. nephronophthisis
E. tuberous sclerosis

153. **A 19-year-old woman was seen by an ophthalmologist for corneal opacities and subsequently referred to the renal clinic for assessment of abnormal renal function. She reported a gradual loss in visual acuity and sensitivity to light. She had no relevant family history.**

    Examination of the abdomen showed hepatomegaly.
    Urinalysis showed blood trace, protein 3+, and glucose 1+.

    Investigations:
serum sodium	138 mmol/L (137–144)
serum potassium	3.1 mmol/L (3.5–4.9)
serum creatinine	92 µmol/L (60–110)
serum phosphate	0.64 mmol/L (0.80–1.45)
serum chloride	115 mmol/L (95–107)

    Ultrasound scan of abdomen showed mild splenomegaly and an enlarged nodular liver. Both kidneys demonstrated increased pyramidal echogenicity and no evidence of hydronephrosis.

    Which is the most appropriate medical management?

    A. captopril
    B. carnitine
    C. cysteamine
    D. nicotinamide
    E. penicillamine

154. **A 28-year-old woman with tuberous sclerosis was reviewed in the renal clinic. She was diagnosed in childhood, having presented with seizures, developmental delay, and skin lesions. She was well and had no symptoms of note. Her medications include levetiracetam and levothyroxine.**

    On examination, her BP was 110/60 mmHg.

    Investigations:
serum creatinine	117 µmol/L (60–110)

    MRI scan of kidneys showed there was progression in the size and number of renal cysts bilaterally. The angiomyolipoma in the upper pole of the right kidney has increased in size. There is a fat-rich mass in the upper pole of the left kidney (31 × 10 mm), indicating a second significant angiomyolipoma. There was no active haemorrhage and no features of renal cell carcinoma.

    Which is the most appropriate next management step?

    A. corticosteroids
    B. embolization
    C. everolimus
    D. sirolimus
    E. tolvaptan

155. A 46-year-old woman was referred by the GP to the renal outpatient clinic. She recently had a CT scan of the abdomen for investigation of abdominal pain and weight loss. She had no urinary symptoms and never had a urinary tract infection. She had a past history of alcohol misuse and chronic pancreatitis. Her current medications included pancreatin supplements and multivitamins.

> On examination, her BP was 130/60 mmHg.
> Urinalysis showed no blood or protein.

Investigations:
serum creatinine	101 µmol/L (60–110)
serum adjusted calcium	2.21 mmol/L (2.20–2.60)
serum parathyroid hormone	11.6 pmol/L (0.9–5.4)
serum amylase	82 U/L (60–180)

Urine culture showed no growth at 5 days.
CT scan of abdomen with contrast showed the pancreas is atrophic, with associated calcification. The left kidney showed clusters of medullary/papillary calcification within three renal pyramids, typical of medullary sponge kidney.

Which is the most appropriate next step in management?

A. cefalexin
B. cinacalcet
C. family screening
D. no further action
E. urine calcium measurement

156. A 34-year-old man was referred to the renal outpatient clinic by his GP with a history of right-sided loin pain. His past history included hypertension, for which he was taking ramipril 5 mg daily. He is estranged from his father but tells you that the latter developed kidney failure in his late forties.

> On examination, enlarged kidneys were palpable bilaterally. His BP was 165/78 mmHg,
> urinalysis showed protein 1+.

Investigations:
serum creatinine	92 µmol/L (60–110)
eGFR	79 mL/min/1.73 m^2 (>60)
urine albumin:creatinine ratio	33.0 mg/mmol (<2.5)

Ultrasound scan of kidneys showed both kidneys measuring >15 cm in size, with four distinct cysts on the right kidney and three distinct cysts on the left.

What is the most likely underlying genetic mutation?

A. *MCKD1*
B. *PKD1*
C. *PKD2*
D. *TSC2*
E. *VHL*

157. A 63-year-old woman with autosomal dominant polycystic kidney disease attended the renal outpatient clinic. She was known to have hypertension and was taking ramipril 5 mg once daily. She reported feeling well, but recent blood tests showed a decline in kidney function.

On examination, she had large palpable kidneys and her BP was 138/75 mmHg.

Urinalysis was negative for blood, protein, glucose, leukocytes, and nitrites.

Investigations:

	Now	Three months ago	Six months ago
serum sodium (mmol/L (137–144))	134	132	132
serum potassium (mmol/L (3.5–4.9))	4.2	4.6	4.3
serum creatinine (µmol/L (60–110))	95	80	65
eGFR (mL/min/1.73 m² (>60))	55	68	87

What is the most important next step in her management?

A. MRI scan of kidneys
B. refer for genetic testing
C. start tolvaptan
D. stop ramipril
E. ultrasound scan of kidneys

158. A 38-year-old man was referred to the renal clinic with an incidental finding of abnormal renal function. He described being fit and healthy, and took no regular medication. He did mention a family history of kidney disease, with his maternal grandfather, uncle, and aunt all suffering from 'kidney problems', although he is unsure of the exact details.

On examination, his BP was 132/68 mmHg.

Urinalysis showed protein 2+.

Investigations:
serum creatinine   163 µmol/L (60–110)
eGFR   45 mL/min/1.73 m² (>60)
urine albumin:creatinine ratio   120 mg/mmol (<2.5)
renal biopsy   (see Fig)

Which of the following is a common feature of this condition?

A. angiofibromata
B. hypokalaemia
C. kidney stones
D. left ventricular hypertrophy
E. seizures

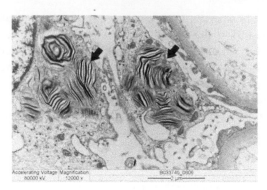

Reproduced with permission from Neves et al, comparative case reports, *BMC Nephrology*, 2017; 18: 157. doi: 10.1186/s12882-017-0571-0.

159. **A 35 year old Afro-Caribbean man with no significant past medical history was assessed as a potential live kidney donor for his friend. He was fit and well and worked as an electrician. He did not smoke and took no regular medications. He had no family history of renal disease.**

   On examination, blood pressure was 136/74 mmHg
   Urinalysis was negative for blood or protein.

   Investigations
   serum creatinine   81 μmol/L
   isotope GFR   105 mL/min/1.73 m^2
   urine albumin:creatinine ratio   1.2 mmol/L (<2.5)
   haemoglobin A1c   36 mmol/L (20–42)
   APOL-1 screen G_0/G_1, "low-risk" renal genotype

   What is the most appropriate advice to give regarding APOL-1 genotype and kidney donation?

   A. Donor APOL-1 genotype is only relevant in the presence of proteinuria
   B. His risk of developing end stage renal disease in his lifetime will increase by 3-4 times post-donation
   C. Kidneys from donors with one APOL-1 high-risk allele have reduced allograft survival compared to donors with no high risk APOL-1 alleles.
   D. Recipient APOL-1 genotype does not affect allograft outcomes.
   E. The APOL-1 high-risk renal genotype is an absolute contra-indication to kidney donation

160. **A 43-year-old Caucasian woman presented to the emergency department with lethargy, nausea, breathlessness, and reduced urine output. There was no history of fevers, cough, rash, abdominal pain, diarrhoea, or joint pain. Her only regular medications included the oral contraceptive pill, which she had been taking for many years.**

On examination, she was afebrile. Her BP was 164/92 mmHg, heart rate 103 beats/min, respiratory rate 23 breaths/min, and oxygen saturations 97% on air.

Urinalysis showed blood 3+, protein 3+.

Investigations:

serum creatinine	773 µmol/L (60–110)
haemoglobin	69 g/L (130–180)
platelet count	82×10^9/L
lactate dehydrogenase	3377 U/L (10–250)
blood film	marked red blood cell fragmentation, polychromasia, and thrombocytopenia
direct Coombs test	negative
ADAMTS 13	50 IU/dL (50–150)
ANCA	negative
serum complement C3	50 mg/dL (65–190)
serum complement C4	8mg/dL (15–50)
renal biopsy	marked endothelial swelling; lumen of small arteries and arterioles obliterated by thrombi

What is the definitive treatment for her condition?

A. eculizumab

B. IVIg

C. plasma exchange

D. prednisolone

E. rituximab

146. C. Early morning urine ACR 40 mg/mmol.

The recipient has X-linked Alport syndrome, which may have been inherited from his mother or due to a sporadic mutation. It is important to establish if his mother is a carrier for the Alport syndrome mutation prior to donation. Donation from Alport syndrome carriers can be considered in appropriately counselled donors aged >45 years in the absence of a family history of deafness, with normal renal function and no proteinuria. Hence a confirmed genetic mutation is not an absolute contraindication to donation. Smoking is strongly discouraged in potential live donors but does not prohibit donation. Persistent non-visible haematuria in donors >40 years of age should be investigated with cystoscopy (and with a renal biopsy if there is concern about glomerular pathology such as a family history of ESRD). National guidelines recommend measured GFR >80 mL/min in potential donors aged 50 or younger. The absolute contraindication to donation in this case would be significant proteinuria in an early morning sample, regardless of whether it has arisen due to the carrier state of Alport syndrome or an alternative glomerular pathology.

British Transplantation Society, The Renal Association (2018). Guidelines for living donor kidney transplantation. Available from: https://bts.org.uk/wp-content/uploads/2018/07/FINAL_LDKT-guidelin es_June-2018.pdf

147. D. Diuretic use

The patient has hypokalaemic metabolic alkalosis (which excludes renal tubular acidosis) and inappropriate renal potassium wasting. The latter makes laxative use less likely, as normal renal physiology would lead to *low* urine potassium. Normal serum magnesium and normal urine calcium levels are not in keeping with Gitelman syndrome (which is characterized by hypomagnesaemia and hypocalciuria). Bartter syndrome is usually diagnosed in childhood or adolescence, and would be unlikely to arise in the fourth decade with a short history of symptoms. Surreptitious diuretic use is often seen in patients trying to lose weight and leads to relative sodium depletion, secondary hyperaldosteronism, and hypokalaemic hypochloraemic metabolic alkalosis. It can be detected on a urine diuretic screen. Although not in frequent clinical use, urine chloride measurement is useful in distinguishing non-renal potassium loss vs a renal potassium wasting syndrome where the renal tubule cannot effectively reabsorb sodium and chloride in response to intravascular depletion.

Khanna A, Kurtzman NA. Metabolic alkalosis. J Nephrol. 2006;19(Suppl 9):S86–96.

148. B. Calcium carbonate.

The renal biopsy shows deposition of oxalate crystals. In this case, renal oxalosis is likely to be related to secondary (enteric) hyperoxaluria due to previous bowel surgery, which may also have contributed to the patient's native renal disease. Management includes lifestyle modification, such as low-oxalate diet (avoiding rhubarb, tea, and beans), and calcium supplements which increase oxalate precipitation within the gut. Methylprednisolone treatment would be used for acute rejection. The BK viral load is negligible. BK nephropathy is generally seen when the viral load is close to 10,000 copies/mL. On light microscopy, PyVAN causes a tubulointerstitial infiltrate and positive SV40 staining. Infliximab would be used for IBD, and amoxicillin for pyelonephritis.

Geraghty R, Wood K, Sayer JA. Calcium oxalate crystal deposition in the kidney: identification, causes and consequences. Urolithiasis. 2020;48(5):377–84.

149. A. Genetic counselling should be offered as part of conception planning.

Mutations in formin (a glomerular actin-regulatory protein) are one of the commonest causes of familial FSGS. Inheritance is autosomal dominant, with variable penetrance. Identification of *any* genetic cause of FSGS has important implications. Immunosuppression is likely to be ineffective in reducing proteinuria and can be withdrawn. Family members may donate if no genetic mutation is found. Recurrent FSGS post-transplant is very rare in patients with *INF2* mutations (<10%); hence adjuvant treatment with rituximab or plasma exchange is not required. There is a 50% risk of offspring being affected; hence genetic counselling should be offered to all patients planning to conceive.

Lovric S, Ashraf S, Tan W, Hildebrandt F. Genetic testing in steroid-resistant nephrotic syndrome: when and how? Nephrol Dial Transplant. 2016;31(11):1802–13.

150. C. Type 1 renal tubular acidosis

The patient has hypokalaemic metabolic acidosis, which excludes Gitelman syndrome (alkalosis) and type 4 renal tubular acidosis (hyperkalaemia). Type 2 proximal renal tubular acidosis (which can include Fanconi syndrome) is caused by defective reabsorption of bicarbonate in the proximal tubule, with mild to moderate acidosis and moderate impairment of urine acidification. Distal (type 1) renal tubular acidosis occurs through failure of acid excretion in the collecting duct and results in a phenotype of severe metabolic acidosis, hypercalciuria, and nephrocalcinosis. Urine pH is usually >6. Type 1 renal tubular acidosis is associated with a number of systemic diseases, including rheumatoid arthritis, Sjögren's syndrome, SLE, dysproteinaemias, and analgesic nephropathy. Treatment is supportive and includes potassium citrate and/or sodium bicarbonate to correct urinary acidification.

Palmer BF, Kelepouris E, Clegg DJ. Renal tubular acidosis and management strategies: a narrative review. Adv Ther. 2021;38(2):949–68.

151. E. *UMOD*.

The family history suggests an autosomal dominant (AD) inheritance, which excludes *COL4A5* (X-linked Alport syndrome) and *NPHP1* (autosomal recessive nephronophthisis). Renal imaging is not consistent with AD polycystic kidney disease. AD tubulointerstitial kidney diseases include uromodulin-, mucin-1-, and renin-associated kidney diseases. Uromodulin (*UMOD*) mutations are commoner than mucin-1 (*MUC1*) mutations and associated with gout. Uromodulin (Tamm–Horsfall protein) is an abundant urinary protein, and possible roles include protection against urinary tract infection and stones. In addition to the monogenic form of inherited kidney disease, UMOD gene variants have also been identified in genome-wide association studies (GWAS) in CKD and hypertension. There is currently no definitive treatment for uromodulin kidney disease beyond supportive management of CKD and gout prophylaxis.

In: J Feehally, J Floege, M Tonelli, eds. *Comprehensive Clinical Nephrology*, 6th edition. St Louis, MO: Elsevier; 2019.

Gast C, Marinaki A, Arenas-Herandez M, *et al*. Autosomal dominant tubulointerstitial kidney disease is the most frequent non polycystic genetic kidney disease. BMC Nephrol. 2018;19:301.

152. D. Nephronophthisis.

Nephronophthisis is an autosomal recessive condition causing cystic kidney disease, with cysts typically seen at the corticomedullary junction. Early manifestations include impaired urine concentration (hyposthenuria), leading to renal salt loss and subsequent polyuria and polydipsia. As renal impairment progresses, these clinical features are countered by fluid retention and hypertension. Nephronophthisis is now known to be caused by mutations in genes encoding ciliary proteins. Extra-renal manifestations include: retinal defects, nystagmus, oculomotor apraxia, cerebellar vermis aplasia, skeletal abnormalities, hepatic fibrosis, and situs inversus. Adrenoleukodystrophy is an X-linked recessive condition with a wide phenotypic range from isolated mild adrenal insufficiency to neurodegenerative complications. It is not associated with kidney disease. The normal 09.00 h cortisol in this case is not consistent with this diagnosis. The radiological appearances do not support the diagnosis of autosomal recessive polycystic kidney disease (enlarged echogenic kidneys with small cysts), medullary sponge kidney (echogenic medullary pyramids ± nephrocalcinosis), or tuberous sclerosis (renal cysts and angiomyolipomata).

In: J Feehally, J Floege, M Tonelli, eds. *Comprehensive Clinical Nephrology*, 6th edition. St Louis, MO: Elsevier, 2019.

153. C. Cysteamine.

This patient has cystinosis, an autosomal recessive storage disease that leads to accumulation of lysosomal cystine as a result of mutations in the transport protein cystinosin. The condition has three clinical forms: nephropathic, intermediate, and adult/benign. In nephropathic cystinosis, Fanconi syndrome, renal failure, growth retardation, rickets, and nephrocalcinosis are common and occur in childhood. Corneal deposition of cystine crystals leads to photophobia and reduced visual acuity. Later complications include hypothyroidism, splenomegaly, diabetes, and pulmonary insufficiency. In intermediate forms of cystinosis, a milder phenotype is observed (as in this case) due to reduced, but not absent, functional protein transport.

Cysteamine reduces cystine levels, by converting cystine to compounds that can exit the lysosome. It can slow the progression of CKD and is available as eye drops to slow corneal crystal deposition. Definitive treatment for cystinosis is renal transplantation, and cysteamine should be continued post-transplant to prevent future renal dysfunction and minimize extra-renal manifestations. Carnitine supplementation may mitigate renal carnitine losses as part of Fanconi syndrome, but is not a definitive treatment for cystinosis.

Cystinuria is unrelated to cystinosis. It is an autosomal recessive disorder due to a gene mutation in a tubular amino acid transporter leading to urinary loss of cystine and other cationic amino acids. It is typically diagnosed in young stone-forming patients. Treatments include penicillamine and captopril.

Nicotinamide can be used in inflammatory skin conditions such as acne. It also decreases sodium-dependent phosphate absorption in the gut and therefore could exacerbate hypophosphataemia.

In: J Feehally, J Floege, M Tonelli, eds. *Comprehensive Clinical Nephrology*, 6th edition. St Louis, MO: Elsevier, 2019.

154. C. Everolimus.

Renal angiomyolipomata (AML) are common in tuberous sclerosis complex (TSC) and, although histologically benign, may cause life-threatening haemorrhage and/or progression to end-stage renal disease. UK guidelines suggest regular (1–2 years) MRI surveillance and treatment of AML measuring >3 cm with mTOR inhibitors. Everolimus is used as first-line treatment of AML measuring >3 cm which show interval growth, and has better therapeutic efficacy than sirolimus, particularly in reducing TSC-AML volume. Sirolimus can also be used but is poorly tolerated. For AML that progress despite treatment with everolimus, embolization can be considered but may accelerate loss of renal function. Acute haemorrhage of renal AML is treated by embolization, corticosteroids, or nephrectomy.

Amin S, Kingswood JC, Bolton PF, *et al*. The UK guidelines for management and surveillance of tuberous sclerosis complex. *QJM*. 2019;112(3):171–82.

Luo C, Zhang YS, Zhang MX, *et al*. Everolimus versus sirolimus for angiomyolipoma associated with tuberous sclerosis complex: a multi-institutional retrospective study in China. *Orphanet J Rare Dis*. 2021;16:299.

155. D. No further action.

This patient's CT scan shows an incidental finding of medullary sponge kidney (MSK). The aetiology of this condition is not well understood but is likely to reflect abnormal renal embryogenesis. It is not usually familial, although a few pedigrees have been reported. It is bilateral in about 70% of cases. Treatment is indicated in the context of: (1) symptomatic stone disease or (2) urinary tract infection. It rarely progresses to CKD and is often found incidentally. It is important to differentiate it from medullary calcification due to hyperparathyroidism or hypercalciuria. This patient has mild secondary hyperparathyroidism, which may be related to vitamin D deficiency due to pancreatic insufficiency and is unlikely to be related to renal calcification.

In: J Feehally, J Floege, M Tonelli, eds. *Comprehensive Clinical Nephrology*, 6th edition. St Louis, MO: Elsevier, 2019.

156. B. *PKD1*.

Enlarged kidneys with multiple bilateral cysts are highly suggestive of autosomal dominant polycystic kidney disease (ADPKD) (see Table 9.1).

Table 9.1 Ravine unified criteria for ultrasonographic diagnosis of ADPKD

Age (years)	Number of cysts
15–39	At least three unilateral or bilateral cysts
40–59	At least two cysts in each kidney
Above 60	At least four cysts in each kidney

Mutations in the *PKD1* gene (short arm chromosome 16) account for 85% of cases of ADPKD. PKD1 mutation is commoner in men and typically causes a more severe phenotype than PKD2 mutation, including: first-degree relative starting renal replacement therapy aged <55 years, early-onset hypertension, enlarged kidneys, loin pain, and haematuria.

Clinical features of other common cystic kidney diseases are summarized in Table 9.2.

Table 9.2 Cytogenetic, pathophysiological, and imaging characteristics of hereditary renal cystic diseases in adults

Condition	Inheritance	Gene, chromosome, protein	Pathophysiological features	Imaging features
Autosomal dominant polycystic kidney disease	Autosomal dominant	*PKD1*, 16p13, polycystin 1 *PKD2*; 4q21, polycystin 2	Renal ciliary dysfunction resulting in increased proliferation of renal tubular epithelium and fluid secretion	Bilateral enlarged kidneys with multiple expansile cysts
Medullary cystic kidney disease	Autosomal dominant	*MCKD1*, 1q21, unknown *MCKD2*, 16p12, uromodulin	Exact pathogenesis uncertain; ciliary dysfunction believed to be secondary to altered interaction between MCKD1 or MCKD2 protein and nephrocystin	Multiple cysts at the corticomedullary junction and in the medulla
Von–Hippel Lindau disease	Autosomal dominant	*VHL*, 3p25-26, pVHL	Upregulation of HIF, with resultant increase in its downstream effectors; derangement of ciliary assembly and mechanosensory function of renal cilium	Multiple, variably sized cysts in both kidneys; multiple interspersed solid and cystic renal cell carcinomas
Tuberous sclerosis complex	Autosomal dominant	*TSC1*, 9q34, hamartin *TSC2*, 16p13, tuberin	Uncontrolled activation of mTOR and its downstream effectors; defects in ciliary function and epithelial cell polarity	Multiple bilateral renal cysts, intermixed with angiomyolipomas

Hateboer N, van Dijk MA, Bogdanova N, *et al*. Exploring the different phenotype of PKD1 and PKD mutations in ADPKD. Comparison of phenotypes of polycystic kidney disease types 1 and 2. European PKD1-PKD2 Study Group. Lancet. 1999;353(9147):103–7.

Pei Y, Obaji J, Dupuis A, *et al*. Ultrasonographic diagnostic criteria for ADPKD: unified criteria for ultrasonographic diagnosis of ADPKD. J Am Soc Nephrol. 2009;20(1):205–12.

Rizk D, Chapman AB. Gene mutations associated with cystic kidney disease. Cystic and inherited kidney diseases. Am J Kidney Dis. 2003;42(6):1305–17.

157. C. Start tolvaptan.

This patient meets criteria for commencing tolvaptan (ADPKD) with CKD stage 2 or 3 and rapidly declining kidney function). Tolvaptan is a vasopressin-2 receptor antagonist that has been shown to slow cyst formation and progression of CKD in patients with ADPKD. Two key tolvaptan trials, TEMPO and REPRISE, recruited patients with eGFR >60 and 25–65 mL/min/1.73 m^2, respectively. Both trials demonstrated a reduced rate of renal decline in the treatment group, with reduced symptom burden and smaller kidney volume, compared to placebo. Side effects were common, however, and were related to aquaresis, for example, excessive thirst, nocturia, and lethargy, as well as liver dysfunction (which usually resolved on discontinuation of tolvaptan).

There is no role for genetic testing or further imaging in this case. Stopping ramipril may lead to a physiological increase in patient's GFR but will not slow her rate of renal progression.

Landmark Nephrology (2019). Landmark trials in ADPKD: close, but no cigar. Available from: https://landmarknephrology.com/topic/adpkd/

National Institute for Health and Care Excellence (2015). Tolvaptan for treating autosomal dominant polycystic kidney disease. Technology appraisal guidance [TA358]. Available from: https://www.nice.org.uk/guidance/ta358

158. D. Left ventricular hypertrophy.

The biopsy image shows a 'zebra body', pathognomonic of Fabry disease. This is an X-linked lysosomal storage disease due to α-galactosidase A (alpha-Gal-A) deficiency. Although men are more commonly affected, heterozygote women can also display features of Fabry disease. Cardiac manifestations are seen in up to 80% of men and can include: concentric left ventricular hypertrophy/hypertrophic cardiomyopathy, myocardial fibrosis, heart failure, coronary artery disease, aortic/mitral valve abnormalities, and conduction abnormalities. Other features of Fabry disease can include: stroke, acroparaesthesiae, telangiectasia and angiokeratomata, abdominal pain, corneal opacities (cornea verticillata), chronic kidney disease, and hearing loss.

Treatment with recombinant enzyme replacement therapy (ERT) and chaperone therapy are available. ERT has been shown to be associated with a small risk of renal and cardiovascular complications but is less effective in patients with established organ damage at the time of starting treatment.

Angiofibromata and seizures are associated with tuberous sclerosis complex. Neither hypokalaemia nor stones are seen in Fabry disease.

Ortiz A, Germain DP, Desnick RJ, et al. Fabry disease revisited: management and treatment recommendations for adult patients. Mol Genet Metab. 2018;123(4):416–27.

van der Veen SJ, Hollak CEM, van Kuilenburg ABP, et al. Developments in the treatment of Fabry disease. J Inherit Metab Dis. 2020;43(5):908–21.

159. Answer: B His risk of developing end stage renal disease in his lifetime will increase by 3-4 times post-donation

Patients of African ancestry with two renal risk variants of the Apoliprotein L1 (APOL-1) gene are known to have a 'high-risk renal genotype' and have an increased lifetime risk of developing end-stage renal disease. Not all patients with a high-risk renal genotype will go on to develop kidney disease however, and an additional "second hit" (eg. hypertension, HIV, COVID-19) is often identified. Although APOL-1 mediated kidney disease is associated with proteinuria, this does not impact upon the interpretation of genotyping.

Kidneys from healthy donors with APOL-1 high-risk renal genotype may have reduced allograft survival compared to kidneys from donors with a low-risk renal genotype, although data are lacking. The APOL-1 genotype of the recipient may also affect transplant outcomes, eg. rejection. Live donors with APOL-1 high-risk renal genotype may suffer an accelerated decline in kidney function following donation, however further research is still ongoing in this area. Although not an absolute contra-indication to proceeding with live donation, many centres would advise caution in younger donors (age <50 years) with APOL-1 high risk renal genotype.

This patient has a low risk renal genotype, which does not further increase his risk of end stage kidney disease post-donation, hence B is the correct answer.

Friedman DJ, Pollak MR. APOL1 Nephropathy: From Genetics to Clinical Applications. Clin J Am Soc Nephrol. 2021 Feb 8;16(2):294–303.

160. A. Eculizumab.

The patient has advanced renal dysfunction, in addition to thrombocytopenia, anaemia, high LDH, and schistocytes on the blood film, in keeping with microangiopathic haemolytic anaemia (MAHA).

The normal ADAMTS13 level, negative pregnancy test, and immunology exclude other possible causes of MAHA and make atypical HUS the most likely diagnosis.

Atypical HUS is a rare complement-mediated disorder leading to thrombotic microangiopathy. Standard of treatment is now with eculizumab, a recombinant monoclonal antibody that inhibits terminal complement activation at the level of C5 protein. Patients require meningococcal vaccination prior to eculizumab treatment, and where treatment cannot be delayed, antibiotic prophylaxis is recommended during the first few weeks of treatment.

George JN, Nester CM. Syndromes of thrombotic microangiopathy. N Engl J Med. 2014;371(7):654–66.

National Institute for Health and Care Excellence (2015). Eculizumab for treating atypical haemolytic uraemic syndrome. Highly specialized technologies guidance [HST1]. Available from: https://www.nice.org.uk/guidance/hst1

Take-Home Messages

1. In patients with ADPKD, *PKD-1* mutations tend to have a more severe phenotype than *PKD-2* mutations. Tolvaptan is recommended for patients with rapidly deteriorating renal function and has been shown to slow cyst formation and progression of CKD.

2. Genetic mutations (as in Alport syndrome) or variants (such as *APOL-1* risk alleles) are not absolute contraindications to live donation, but each patient requires an individualized risk assessment.

3. Patients of African ancestry with two renal risk variants of the *APOL-1* gene are known to have a 'high-risk renal genotype' and have an increased lifetime risk of developing end-stage renal disease.

4. Mutations in formin are one of the commonest causes of familial FSGS. Inheritance is autosomal dominant, with variable penetrance. Recurrent FSGS post-transplant is very rare in patients with *INF2* mutations (<10%).

5. Many rare renal disorders have important extra-renal manifestations, for example, Fabry disease (cardiac), tuberous sclerosis complex (neurological), cystinosis (ophthalmic).

6. Features of Fabry disease can include: stroke, acroparaesthesiae, telangiectasia and angiokeratomata, abdominal pain, corneal opacities (cornea verticillata), chronic kidney disease, left ventricular hypertrophy, and hearing loss.

7. Complex acid–base disturbances can be analysed by differentiating between acidosis and alkalosis, bearing in mind discriminating features of different conditions (e.g. low magnesium in Gitelman syndrome, nephrocalcinosis in distal RTA, etc.).

8. Definitive treatment for cystinosis is renal transplantation, and cysteamine should be continued post-transplant to prevent future renal dysfunction and minimize the risk of extra-renal manifestations.

9. Uromodulin (*UMOD*) mutations are commoner than mucin-1 (*MUC1*) mutations and are associated with gout. There is currently no definitive treatment for *UMOD* mutations.

10. Atypical HUS is a complement-mediated disorder leading to TMA. Standard of treatment is now with eculizumab.

161. **A 45-year-old woman was seen in the low clearance clinic for renal replacement therapy planning, the patient opted for peritoneal dialysis as the modality of choice and a PD catheter was inserted laparoscopically. Two days after the procedure, the patient presented to the renal nurse with fever and abdominal pain.**

   Investigations:
   cell count of dialysate   1300 leukocytes/µL and 300 erythrocytes/µL
   methicillin-sensitive *Staphylococcus aureus* grown in effluent cultures

   Which intervention is most likely to prevent early post-procedural infection?

   A. catheter design
   B. catheter insertion technique
   C. exit site care
   D. systemic prophylactic antibiotic
   E. nasal *S. aureus* eradication

162. **A 72-year-old man on CAPD for 2 years was brought to emergency department by his neighbours due to deteriorating health. He complained of lower abdominal pain for the past 3 days.**

   On examination, his temperature was 38.2°C and his BP was 122/70 mmHg. He had lower abdominal tenderness.

   Investigations:
   Abdominal X-ray showed free air.

   What would be the next appropriate step?

   A. CT scan of abdomen
   B. dialysate sample cell count and culture
   C. empirical antibiotics
   D. PD catheter removal
   E. peritoneal lavage

Best of Five MCQs for the European Specialty Examination in Nephrology. Shafi Malik, Oxford University Press.
© Oxford University Press 2024. DOI: 10.1093/oso/9780192844163.003.0019

163. **A 41-year-old man on CAPD for the past year presents to the PD unit with a 2-day history of new-onset abdominal pain.**

    Physical examination revealed generalized tenderness in the abdomen and rebound was positive. The catheter exit site was clean.

    Investigations:
    effluent cell count   5200 leukocytes/μL; samples were sent for Gram staining and cultures

    What would be the next best management step?
    A. IP cefazolin and IP ceftazidime
    B. IP cefazolin and oral fluconazole
    C. IP gentamicin and oral ciprofloxacin
    D. IP gentamicin and oral fluconazole
    E. IP vancomycin and oral amoxicillin/clavulanate

164. **A 35-year-old man on automated peritoneal dialysis for 6 months was managed with the help of a kinetic modelling software integrated into his APD machine. A substantial decrease in ultrafiltration volumes was detected by the software, and a telephone consultation with the patient revealed good inflow, but delayed outflow time.**

    Which one of the following is the most likely cause of the impaired outflow?
    A. catheter kink
    B. catheter migration
    C. constipation
    D. intraluminal fibrin
    E. omental wrap

165. **A 60-year-old woman on peritoneal dialysis for the past 9 years was admitted to hospital due to recurrent abdominal pain associated with intermittent nausea and vomiting. She was found to have reduced ultrafiltration volumes and poor solute clearances.**

    Investigations:
    effluent cell count   52 leukocytes/μL
    effluent culture   no growth

    CT scan of the abdomen (see Fig).

    What is the most likely diagnosis in this patient?
    A. benign peritoneal fibrosis
    B. bowel cancer
    C. culture-negative peritonitis
    D. encapsulating peritoneal sclerosis
    E. inflammatory bowel disease

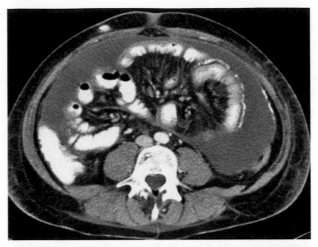

Reproduced with permission from Anniek Vlijm, Joost van Schuppen, Armand B. G. N. Lamers, Dirk G. Struijk, Raymond T. Krediet, *NDT Plus*, Volume 4, Issue 5, October 2011, Pages 281–284, https://doi.org/10.1093/ndtplus/sfr068.

166. A 30-year-old woman with ESRD was started on PD recently. At routine follow-up, metabolic parameters were checked.

	Before PD	Three months after PD
Fasting glucose (mmol/L)	5	6.6
LDL-cholesterol (mmol/L)	6.6	8.3
HDL-cholesterol (mmol/L)	2.5	1.9
Triglyceride (mmol/L)	9.1	12.5

What would explain the hyperglycaemia and dyslipidaemia?

A. diabetes mellitus

B. familial hypercholesterolaemia

C. glucose-containing dialysis solutions

D. metabolic syndrome

E. non-compliance

167. **An 85-year-old woman on CAPD for 2 years gradually became anuric and fluid-overloaded, with lower limb oedema. Her current CAPD prescription was three exchanges with a 1.36% glucose-containing 2 L solution and one overnight exchange with 2 L icodextrin, 8 L daily in total. The patient's body surface area was 1.65 m². A peritoneal equilibration test showed a slow transporter status and her Kt/V was 1.5.**

    What is the most appropriate prescription for the patient?

    A. one 1.36% 2 L solution, two 2.27% 2 L solutions, and one overnight icodextrin
    B. switch modality to haemodialysis
    C. three 1.36% 2 L solutions, one 2.27% 2.5 L solution, and one overnight icodextrin
    D. three 2.27% 2 L solutions and one overnight icodextrin
    E. two 1.36% 2 L solutions, one 2.27% 2 L solution, and one overnight icodextrin

168. **A 40-year-old woman on CAPD underwent an annual peritoneal equilibration test. At 4 hours, peritoneal equilibration test results showed a dialysate:plasma (D/P) creatinine concentration ratio of 0.57.**

    Which of the following is the membrane transporter status of this patient?

    A. average
    B. high
    C. high average
    D. low
    E. low average

169. **A 23-year-old man with end-stage renal disease due to IgA nephropathy was due to be established on PD. He had a significant daily urine output.**

    On examination, his BP was 156/94 mmHg and he had lower limb oedema. He wanted to use automated peritoneal dialysis.

    What would be the optimal prescription for this patient?

    A. four 2-hour exchanges using two 1.36% solutions, 8 L daily
    B. four 2-hour exchanges using one 1.36% and one 2.27% solution, 8 L daily
    C. four 2-hour exchanges using one 2.27% solution and daytime icodextrin, 10 L daily
    D. four 2-hour exchanges using one 2.27% and one 3.86% solution, 8 L daily
    E. five 2-hour exchanges using one 2.27% and one 3.86%, 10 L daily

170. **A 40-year-old woman was recently started on CAPD with four exchanges using a 1.36% glucose-containing solution including acidic pH and standard-glucose degradation products. Two weeks later, she complained of a considerable amount of inflow pain. There were no problems with inflow and outflow volumes.**

What would be the next best step?

A. 1.36% solution exchanges including neutral-pH and low-glucose degradation products
B. check the catheter for kinks
C. check the catheter for intraluminal debris
D. modality switch to haemodialysis
E. switch to automated peritoneal dialysis

171. **A 60-year-old woman with ESRD due to PKD was seen in the low clearance clinic to discuss the choice of modality. Her BMI was 31.2 kg/m². She had a history of an uncomplicated caesarean section. Five days before her appointment, she presented to emergency department with mild abdominal pain and a CT scan of the abdomen confirmed acute diverticulitis, in addition to renal and liver cysts. She was started on appropriate antibiotics and responded well. She is also keen on a renal transplant and has a potential live donor.**

Which modality would you recommend?

A. conservative care
B. haemodialysis because of the history of abdominal operation
C. haemodialysis because of the obesity
D. haemodialysis since PD is contraindicated in patients with PKD
E. PD after resolution of the diverticulitis

172. **A 70-year-old man with ESRD due to obesity-associated FSGS was on maintenance haemodialysis. He had multiple failed tunnelled venous dialysis catheters and arteriovenous fistulae. He was advised a modality change to PD. His BMI was 41.4 kg/m², and he had multiple skinfolds on his abdomen.**

What PD catheter would you recommend?

A. extended catheter with an upper abdominal exit site
B. extended catheter with a presternal exit site
C. standard Tenckhoff catheter with a laterally directed exit site
D. swan neck catheter
E. Toronto Western catheter

173. **A 75-year-old man living in a care home due to hemiparesis has been on assisted APD. A green-coloured discharge from the catheter exit site was noted on routine examination. An ultrasound scan of the abdomen showed no signs of tunnel infection.**

    On examination, his temperature was 36.5°C and there was no abdominal tenderness.

    Investigations:
    exit site swab   profuse growth of Pseudomonas species

    What would be the next appropriate step?

    A. amoxicillin
    B. ceftazidime
    C. ciprofloxacin
    D. tobramycin
    E. vancomycin

174. **A 40-year-old woman on PD for 2 months presented to the PD nurse with erythema and localized pain on her abdomen. On examination, she had tenderness over the subcutaneous PD catheter tunnel. Cell count of the dialysate revealed only 5 leukocytes/µL. Specimens were taken from both the dialysate and the exit site for Gram staining and cultures. Gram staining from the exit site showed Gram-positive cocci.**

    Which would be the best first-line antibiotic of choice?

    A. cefalexin
    B. ciprofloxacin
    C. linezolid
    D. rifampicin
    E. vancomycin

175. **A 60-year-old man with ESRD was seen in the low clearance clinic for discussion of the dialysis modality. He had good residual renal function with a daily urine volume of 2 L, and his last eGFR was 11 mL/min/1.73 m^2.**

    On physical examination, his BP was 125/80 mmHg and he was euvolaemic.

    Which modality would you recommend in order to preserve his residual renal function?

    A. home haemodialysis
    B. in-centre haemodialysis
    C. nocturnal haemodialysis
    D. peritoneal dialysis
    E. satellite unit haemodialysis

176. An 80-year-old man had been on assisted **PD** performed by family members uneventfully for 3 years, with regular follow-up. During the outbreak of **COVID-19** in 2020, both the patient and his family expressed their reluctance to come to hospital for follow-up.

Which component of a remote monitoring programme would be a challenge for this patient?

A. burden on family members
B. home-based treatment
C. maintaining dialysis supplies
D. monitoring of RRF
E. remote visits with telemedicine

177. A 60-year-old woman on **PD** for 4 years presented to her **PD** nurse with weight gain and bilateral lower limb oedema which gradually increased over 3 months. The Kt/V was 1.9. The patient was diagnosed with ultrafiltration failure. Mini- and standard peritoneal equilibration tests revealed that the 1-hour ultrafiltration was 20% of the total ultrafiltration volume.

Which component of the peritoneum could be responsible for the ultrafiltration failure in this patient?

A. interstitium
B. large pores
C. mesothelial cell layer
D. small pores
E. ultra-small pores

178. A 50-year-old man on **CAPD** has been on the following treatment regimen: three exchanges with a 1.36% glucose-containing solution and an overnight icodextrin exchange, 8 L in total daily. His urine volume gradually decreased and he became slightly fluid-overloaded. The Kt/V was 2.0. The dialysis prescription was changed to two exchanges with a 1.36% glucose-containing solution, one exchange with a 2.27% glucose-containing solution, and an overnight icodextrin exchange, 8 L daily in total.

In 60–90 minutes of a dwell with the 2.27% glucose-containing solution, which serum electrolyte abnormality would be expected in this patient?

A. hypokalaemia
B. hyperkalaemia
C. hypomagnesaemia
D. hyponatraemia
E. hypernatraemia

179. **A 60-year-old woman had been on CAPD. In the last 2 months, she began to notice a subcutaneous swelling in the peri-catheter area, accompanied by a gradual decrease in ultrafiltration volumes. On examination, there was moderate subcutaneous oedema around the catheter. Imaging modalities confirmed a dialysate leak.**

How would you manage this patient?

A. continue CAPD and reduce the total daily exchange volume

B. continue CAPD and add an extra daytime exchange

C. modality switch to haemodialysis

D. refer for surgery

E. switch to CCPD

180. **A 50-year-old man on CAPD unintentionally lost 15% body weight over the last 6 months. His prescription was three exchanges with a 1.36% glucose-containing 2 L solution and an overnight icodextrin 2 L exchange, 8 L daily in total.**

On examination, he was euvolaemic and his BMI was 19 kg/m².

Investigations:
serum albumin   28 g/L (37–49)
Kt/V   1.6

Peritoneal equilibration test demonstrated a slow transporter status.

What should be the next management step?

A. continue the current CAPD regime

B. modality switch to haemodialysis

C. three exchanges with 1.36% solution and overnight icodextrin, 10 L daily in total

D. two exchanges with 1.36% solution, one exchange with 2.27% solution, and overnight icodextrin, 8 L daily in total

E. two exchanges with 1.36% solution, one exchange with an amino acid-containing solution, and one overnight icodextrin exchange, 10 L daily in total

161. D. Systemic prophylactic antibiotic.

Systemic administration of a prophylactic antibiotic immediately prior to catheter insertion is the most critical step for prevention of PD-related peritonitis. First-generation cephalosporins, such as cefazolin, are still commonly used due to concerns of vancomycin resistance, although it may be less effective than vancomycin. Catheter design and insertion technique have not been shown to affect infection-related outcomes. Exit site care with topical antibiotics is recommended to reduce exit site infections. The significance of nasal *S. aureus* carriage is still under debate.

Li PK, Chow KM, Cho Y, *et al*. ISPD peritonitis guideline recommendations: 2022 update on prevention and treatment. Perit Dial Int. 2022 Mar;42(2):110–153.

162. B. Dialysate sample cell count and culture.

This is most likely PD related peritonitis with systemic inflammatory features in an elderly patient. Free air on X-ray is not surprising, since all PD patients have some free air in their abdomen. The first approach to any patient on PD with suspected peritonitis should include early sampling of the dialysis effluent (after a minimum 2-hour dwell) and testing for cell count differential, Gram staining, and cultures. After sampling, the patient must be started on intraperitoneal or intravenous antibiotics, according to International Society for Peritoneal Dialysis guidelines, which recommend empirical Gram-positive and Gram-negative cover, with a first-generation cephalosporin or vancomycin for Gram-positive cover and a third-generation cephalosporin or an aminoglycoside for Gram-negative cover or monotherapy with a fourth-generation cephalosporin.

Li PK, Chow KM, Cho Y, *et al*. ISPD peritonitis guideline recommendations: 2022 update on prevention and treatment. Perit Dial Int. 2022 Mar;42(2):110–153.

163. A. IP cefazolin and IP ceftazidime.

Immediately after appropriate sampling of dialysis effluent, empirical antibiotics must be administered covering Gram-positive and Gram-negative organisms. Intraperitoneal delivery is preferred unless the patient has features of sepsis. Gram-positive organisms would be covered by vancomycin or a first-generation cephalosporin (i.e. cefazolin), whereas third-generation cephalosporins (i.e. ceftazidime) or aminoglycosides should be chosen to cover Gram-negatives. A fourth-generation cephalosporin could be used as monotherapy. Although vancomycin would be preferred for Gram-positive cover, in the given options, vancomycin with amoxicillin/clavulanate would not be recommended. However, vancomycin along with ciprofloxacin for Gram-negative cover would be appropriate.

Li PK, Chow KM, Cho Y, *et al*. ISPD peritonitis guideline recommendations: 2022 update on prevention and treatment. Perit Dial Int. 2022 Mar;42(2):110–153.

Best of Five MCQs for the European Specialty Examination in Nephrology. Shafi Malik, Oxford University Press.
© Oxford University Press 2024. DOI: 10.1093/oso/9780192844163.003.0020

164. C. Constipation.

Outflow failure is indicative of catheter flow dysfunction and constipation is the commonest cause. Distension of the rectosigmoid colon can block the catheter holes or displace the tip. Intraluminal fibrin, catheter kinks, and migration should be considered once constipation is ruled out. Omental wrap is a rare cause of catheter malfunction and is only considered after the above causes are excluded.

Crabtree JH, Shrestha BM, Chow KM et al. Creating and maintaining optimal peritoneal dialysis access in the adult patient: 2019 update. Perit Dial Int. 2019;39(5):414–36.

Jheng JS, Chang CT, Huang CC. Omental wrapping of a peritoneal dialysis catheter. Kidney Int. 2012;82(7):827.

165. D. Encapsulating peritoneal sclerosis.

Encapsulating peritoneal sclerosis (EPS) is a rare complication seen in patients on PD long term. Length of PD treatment (usually over 5 years) and multiple episodes of peritonitis are risk factors. It is characterized by intraperitoneal inflammation and fibrosis, leading to encapsulation of the bowels. Patients present with symptoms of intermittent obstruction. EPS must be distinguished from benign peritoneal fibrosis, which can occur in PD patients. Benign peritoneal fibrosis is often clinically silent and occur without radiological signs. For culture-negative peritonitis, the PD effluent should have >100 leukocytes/μL.

Augustine T, Brown PW, Davies SD, Summers AM, Wilkie ME. Encapsulating peritoneal sclerosis: clinical significance and implications. Nephron Clin Pract. 2009;111:c149–54.

166. C. Glucose-containing dialysis solutions.

Several factors affect glucose and lipid metabolism in PD patients. The main driver is the glucose content in dialysis solutions. Absorption of glucose from the dialysate not only causes hyperglycaemia and weight gain, but also constitutes new substrates for lipid synthesis, thereby causing dyslipidaemia. This is not diabetes or familial hypercholesterolaemia. There is insufficient information to diagnose metabolic syndrome.

Attman PO, Samuelsson O, Johansson AC, et al. Dialysis modalities and dyslipidemia. Kidney Int Suppl. 2003;(84):S110–12.

167. C. Three 1.36% 2 L solutions, one 2.27% 2.5 L solution, and one overnight icodextrin.

In order to achieve adequate solute clearances in an anuric PD patient, the number and volume of exchanges should be incrementally increased. In this patient with a body surface area below 1.7 m^2 and a slow transporter status, increasing the CAPD volume to 10–12.5 L daily or switching to automated peritoneal dialysis would be recommended. Before switching modality, other options should be exhausted.

Rippe B. Peritoneal Dialysis: Principles, Techniques, and Adequacy. In: Feehally J, Floege J, Tonelli M, Johnson RJ, eds. *Comprehensive Clinical Nephrology*, 6th edition. Edinburgh, UK: Elsevier, 2019; pp. 1103–1113.

168. E. Low average.

The D/P ratio for creatinine in the peritoneal equilibration test at 4 hours helps to categorize patients into four groups, according to their membrane transporter status: low (0.34 to <0.50), low average (0.50 to <0.65), high average (0.65 to <0.81), and high (0.81 to 1.03). A high membrane transporter status is also referred to as fast, and a low membrane transporter status as slow.

Rippe B. Peritoneal Dialysis: Principles, Techniques, and Adequacy. In: Feehally J, Floege J, Tonelli M, Johnson RJ, eds. *Comprehensive Clinical Nephrology*, 6th edition. Edinburgh, UK: Elsevier, 2019; pp. 1103–1113.

169. A. Four 2-hour exchanges using two 1.36% solutions, 8 L daily.

In automated peritoneal dialysis, a cycler used overnight for 8–10 hours facilitates large-volume exchanges. During daytime, patients can perform additional long dwells using icodextrin if adequate solute clearance and ultrafiltration are required (wet day). When being established on automated peritoneal dialysis, a patient with an average weight usually starts with 2 L exchanges, with a minimum of 8–10 L daily. Since the patient has good residual renal function, additional daytime exchanges would not be necessary. If additional ultrafiltration is needed, 2.27% glucose solutions may be used. High-glucose-containing solutions are used with caution due to the risk of developing membrane failure.

Rippe B. Peritoneal Dialysis: Principles, Techniques, and Adequacy. In: Feehally J, Floege J, Tonelli M, Johnson RJ, eds. *Comprehensive Clinical Nephrology*, 6th edition. Edinburgh, UK: Elsevier, 2019; pp. 1103–1113.

Brown EA, Peter G Blake, Neil Boudville, *et al.* International Society for Peritoneal Dialysis practice recommendations: prescribing high-quality goal-directed peritoneal dialysis. Perit Dial Int. 2020;40(3):244–53.

170. A. 1.36% solution exchanges including neutral-pH and low-glucose degradation products.

Biocompatibility is an important aspect of peritoneal dialysis solutions. Use of neutral-pH and low-glucose degradation product-containing solutions is associated with better RRF, increased urine volumes, and reduced inflow pain. If available, biocompatible solutions should be of choice in all patients on peritoneal dialysis.

Cho Y, Johnson DW, Badve SV, *et al.* The impact of neutral-pH peritoneal dialysates with reduced glucose degradation products on clinical outcomes in peritoneal dialysis patients. Kidney Int. 2013;84(5):969–79.

171. E. PD after resolution of the diverticulitis.

A history of an uncomplicated abdominal surgery is not a contraindication to PD, provided that there are no intra-abdominal adhesions. Mild obesity is also not a contraindication. PD can be performed in patients with PKD, but caution is warranted during catheter insertion. Active diverticulitis is a contraindication; however, after resolution of active inflammation, the patient can start PD safely. PD is also a good modality as a bridge to transplantation.

Blake PG, Quinn RR, Oliver MJ. Peritoneal dialysis and the process of modality selection. Perit Dial Int. 2013;33(3):233–41.

172. B. Extended catheter with presternal exit site.

In patients with severe obesity and multiple skinfolds on the abdomen, an extended catheter with a presternal exit site should be chosen for insertion. The subcutaneous fat layer is relatively thin in the presternal area, which minimizes catheter dysfunction. A presternal exit site must be considered for patients with intestinal stomas, severe obesity, multiple abdominal skinfolds, intestinal stomas, or incontinence.

Crabtree JH, Shrestha BM, Chow KM, *et al.* Creating and maintaining optimal peritoneal dialysis access in the adult patient: 2019 update. Perit Dial Int. 2019;39(5):414–36.

173. C. Ciprofloxacin.

Exit site infections (ESIs) can be caused by various organisms. When treating ESIs, empirical antibiotics must cover *Staphylococcus* species. A green-coloured discharge from the exit site is usually associated with *Pseudomonas* infections. These infections are difficult to treat and require prolonged courses. Oral fluoroquinolones are recommended as the first-line choice. However, due to concerns about resistance, these infections are generally treated with two antibiotics. As the patient is clinically well, ciprofloxacin would be a good initial choice.

Szeto CC, Li PK, Johnson DW *et al.* ISPD catheter-related infection recommendations: 2017 update. Perit Dial Int. 2017;37(2):141–54.

174. A. Cefalexin.

Tunnel infection usually presents with concomitant exit site infection. It may manifest as erythema, induration, oedema, or tenderness, or it may be clinically occult and diagnosed by ultrasound. Empirical antibiotic therapy must cover *Staphylococcus aureus* with penicillinase-resistant penicillin or first-generation cephalosporins, provided that the patient has no history of infection or colonization with methicillin-resistant *S. aureus* (MRSA) or *Pseudomonas* species. Vancomycin and linezolid should be of choice when MRSA is suspected. Ciprofloxacin must be part of an anti-pseudomonal regimen.

Szeto CC, Li PK, Johnson DW *et al.* ISPD catheter-related infection recommendations: 2017 update. Perit Dial Int. 2017;37(2):141–54.

175. D. Peritoneal dialysis.

RRF improves survival in patients with ESRD. RRF has been shown to be associated with reductions in BP and left ventricular volumes, higher haemoglobin levels, and better nutritional status. Preservation of RRF can be better achieved on PD than on haemodialysis, and RRF is closely associated with technique survival in PD.

Marrón B, Remón C, Pérez-Fontán M, Quirós P, Ortíz A. Benefits of preserving residual renal function in peritoneal dialysis. Kidney Int Suppl. 2008 Apr;(108):S42–51.

176. E. Remote visits with telemedicine.

During the COVID-19 pandemic, home-based dialysis modalities conferred an advantage, compared to in-centre haemodialysis, due to social distancing requirements. Nonetheless, home dialysis can create some challenges such as burden on family members and problems of monitoring of RRF. For this patient, an uneventful course of assisted peritoneal dialysis suggests that these potential setbacks may not be an obstacle to monitoring. However, remote visits with telemedicine can still be an issue, since fragile and elderly patients may experience difficulty with expressing their problems clearly.

Cozzolino M, Piccoli GB, Ikizler TA, *et al.* The COVID-19 infection in dialysis: are home-based renal replacement therapies a way to improve patient management? J Nephrol. 2020;33(4):629–31.

177. E. Ultra-small pores.

The peritoneal membrane consists of three layers: capillary wall, interstitium, and mesothelial cell layer. The capillary wall has a system consisting of three pores with different roles in solute and water clearances: large, small, and ultra-small (aquaporin-1). True UF failure constitutes a significant barrier to peritoneal dialysis practice. Transcapillary movement of free water across ultra-small pores is responsible for nearly half of the UF volume, and loss of its function leads to type 2 UF failure (low osmotic conductance to glucose), which can be estimated by comparing the first-hour UF with the total UF. A ratio of 0.26 or less has been found to be associated with impaired aquaporin-1 function.

Teitelbaum I. Ultrafiltration failure in peritoneal dialysis: a pathophysiologic approach. Blood Purif. 2015;39(1–3):70–3.

178. E. Hypernatraemia.

Glucose is an intermediate-size osmolyte, with limited osmotic efficacy across small pores in the peritoneum. However, it has 100% efficacy when it comes to the ultra-small pore system (aquaporin-1). As a result, free water transport through aquaporin-1 channels creates significant sodium sieving, which can cause hypernatraemia in the first 60–90 minutes of a dwell with high-glucose-containing solutions.

Rippe B. Peritoneal Dialysis: Principles, Techniques, and Adequacy. In: Feehally J, Floege J, Tonelli M, Johnson RJ, eds. *Comprehensive Clinical Nephrology*, 6th edition. Edinburgh, UK: Elsevier, 2019; pp. 1103–1113.

Trinh E, Perl J. The patient receiving automated peritoneal dialysis with volume overload. Clin J Am Soc Nephrol. 2018;13(11):1732–4.

179. E. Switch to CCPD.

Dialysate leak is a significant non-infectious complication of PD, which can be early or late. Late leaks are generally seen within 2 years of PD initiation, especially in patients on CAPD. Abdominal wall weakness and increased intra-abdominal pressure are important risk factors. Rest from CAPD for 1–3 weeks is the optimal treatment. During this resting period, patients can be switched to APD, CCPD, or temporary haemodialysis. Daytime exchanges should not be added to the prescription if automated PD is preferred.

Leblanc M, Ouimet D, Pichette V. Dialysate leaks in peritoneal dialysis. Semin Dial. 2001;14(1):50–4.

180. E. Two exchanges with 1.36% solution, one exchange with an amino acid-containing solution, and one overnight icodextrin exchange, 10 L daily in total.

Malnutrition is more frequent in PD patients. Low albumin, low BMI, and unintentional weight loss of >5% over 3 months or >10% over 6 months are diagnostic of malnutrition. All malnourished patients without a rapid transporter status should be treated with increased dialysis, thereby improving appetite. Exchange with an amino acid-containing solution may help increase appetite further; it has also been shown to improve the nutritional status.

Kicbalo T, Holotka J, Habura I, Pawlaczyk K. Nutritional status in peritoneal dialysis: nutritional guidelines, adequacy and the management of malnutrition. Nutrients. 2020;12(6):1715.

Take-Home Messages

1. Systemic antibiotic prophylaxis immediately prior to catheter insertion is the most critical step for the prevention of post-procedure peritonitis.
2. When PD peritonitis is suspected, the PD effluent should be sampled after a minimum 2-hour dwell and samples sent for cell count, differential, Gram staining, and cultures. Following this, the patient must be started on empirical antibiotics to cover Gram-positive and Gram-negative organisms.
3. Outflow failure is indicative of catheter flow dysfunction; constipation is the commonest cause.
4. Glucose-containing dialysis solutions can cause hyperglycaemia, weight gain, and dyslipidaemia.
5. The number and volume of exchanges should be incrementally increased to achieve adequate solute clearances and ultrafiltration.
6. The peritoneal equilibration test categorizes patients according to the transport status of the peritoneal membrane.
7. A history of uncomplicated abdominal surgery, mild obesity, and PKD are not contraindications to PD.

8. The RRF is associated with improved outcomes. It leads to better BP control, volume status, and nutritional status, and higher haemoglobin levels. It is also associated with technique survival in PD.

9. Malnutrition is more frequent in PD patients, compared to those on haemodialysis; increasing the dialysis prescription and exchange with an amino acid-containing solution can help.

10. Transcapillary movement of free water across ultra-small pores is responsible for nearly half of the ultrafiltration volume, and loss of its function leads to type 2 ultrafiltration failure

181. **A 22-year-old man with CKD of unknown aetiology was admitted a
week earlier with uraemic symptoms. At the time of admission, he had
a pericardial friction rub. A transthoracic echocardiogram showed left
ventricular hypertrophy and no evidence of pericardial effusion. He was
discharged home after three sessions of haemodialysis.**

    He presented 3 days later as an emergency with sudden-onset shortness of breath. His
    BP was 80/40 mmHg, and the JVP was 5 cm above the sternal angle. His heart sounds
    were quiet and there was no pericardial rub.

    Investigations:
    Chest X ray showed cardiomegaly.

    What is the most appropriate step in his management?

    A. continuous renal replacement therapy
    B. echocardiography
    C. fluid resuscitation
    D. haemodialysis
    E. peritoneal dialysis

182. **You are asked by the staff nurse on the dialysis unit to see a 70-year-old
man who has been on maintenance haemodialysis for about 6 months
with a tunnelled left internal jugular venous catheter. For the past
2 weeks or so, there have been repeated arterial alarms with low flow
rates during dialysis, with the pre-pump arterial pressure dropping
below 250 mmHg at a blood flow of >300 mL/min. His monthly
Kt/V was 0.9. Clinical examination was unremarkable.**

    What is the most likely diagnosis?

    A. catheter displacement
    B. central venous thrombosis
    C. intraluminal clot
    D. kinked catheter
    E. pericatheter fibrin sheath

Best of Five MCQs for the European Specialty Examination in Nephrology. Shafi Malik, Oxford University Press.
© Oxford University Press 2024. DOI: 10.1093/oso/9780192844163.003.0021

183. At your satellite dialysis unit, it was brought to your attention that four in-centre haemodialysis patients have turned positive for hepatitis C serology during routine 6-monthly surveillance for viral infections.

What would be the most appropriate step to prevent further spread of hepatitis C?

A. continue current dialysis arrangements
B. prophylactic direct-acting antiviral agents for all in-centre patients
C. separate dialysis facility for HCV-positive patients
D. separate RO water lines for HCV-positive patients
E. strict universal precautions in the dialysis facility

184. A 62-year-old man had recently been initiated on haemodialysis. His pre-dialysis BP was 140/90 mmHg, and his BP rose to 180/90 mmHg after 60 minutes of dialysis treatment. His interdialytic weight gain was 2 kg and 500 mL of fluid had been removed so far. He was on optimal dosing of amlodipine, clonidine, and metoprolol to control his BP and had taken all his antihypertensives 3 hours prior to his haemodialysis.

What modifications would you make, based on the dialysability of antihypertensives?

A. replace amlodipine with enalapril
B. replace amlodipine with nifedipine
C. replace clonidine with prazosin
D. replace metoprolol with atenolol
E. replace metoprolol with carvedilol

185. **A 27-year-old man with a history of IgA nephropathy presented with uraemic symptoms and fluid overload. He was initiated on haemodialysis through a temporary right internal jugular venous catheter. He was dialysed for 3 hours, with a blood flow of 200 mL/min and a dialysate flow of 500 mL/min. His BP was stable during dialysis and 1 L ultrafiltration was done.**

He complained of mild headache after dialysis but was otherwise well. After 2 hours or so, he developed agitation followed by a generalized seizure. A diagnosis of dialysis disequilibrium syndrome was made.

Investigations:

serum urea	70 mmol/L (2.5–7.0)
serum creatinine	1464 µmol/L (60–110)
serum bicarbonate	7 mmol/L (20–28)
serum adjusted calcium	1.6 mmol/L (2.20–2.60)

What steps could have been taken during dialysis to reduce the risk of dialysis disequilibrium syndrome?

A. increase blood flow and dialysate flow
B. longer treatment time
C. reduce blood flow and dialysate flow
D. reduce dialysate sodium
E. reduce ultrafiltration volume

186. **A 72-year-old man who has been on regular thrice-weekly haemodialysis through his right radiocephalic AV fistula for the past 10 years presents to you with a history of right shoulder pain associated with pain and paraesthesiae in the right hand. He gives no history of trauma. Findings from a nerve conduction study were consistent with a diagnosis of carpal tunnel syndrome. He has no residual renal function.**

What modification to his dialysis prescription is likely to benefit him?

A. increase blood and dialysate flow
B. increase the frequency of haemodialysis and switch to a high-flux dialyser
C. increase the frequency of haemodialysis and use a low-flux dialyser with a larger surface area
D. switch to haemodiafiltration
E. switch to peritoneal dialysis

187. **A 72-year-old gentleman with ESRD on thrice-weekly maintenance haemodialysis had a Kt/V between 1.4 and 1.6 since initiation of haemodialysis. He started dialysis with a tunnelled dialysis catheter and then had a right radiocephalic fistula, which has been used for 2 years. The last two single-pool Kt/Vs have remained below 1.0. Recirculation studies showed recirculation of 22%.**

   What is the most appropriate next step in management?

   A. AVF angiography
   B. duplex ultrasound of AVF
   C. pulse augmentation test
   D. spaced-out arterial and venous needles
   E. tunnelled dialysis catheter

188. **A 46-year-old gentleman on haemodialysis for 5 years via a left radiocephalic fistula presents with a history of multiple cord-like swellings over the arteriovenous fistula tract that have been gradually increasing in size over the past year.**

   On inspection, there are three aneurysms along the arteriovenous fistula. There is no thinning of overlying skin, necrotic skin, tenderness, or redness over the sites.

   Which manoeuvre is likely to help establish the aetiology of the aneurysms?

   A. Allen's test
   B. arm elevation test
   C. Nicoladoni–Israel–Branham sign
   D. pulse augmentation test
   E. sequential occlusion test

189. **A 26-year-old lady on regular thrice-weekly haemodialysis presents to the emergency department with sudden-onset giddiness and diaphoresis. She missed her last dialysis session. An ECG done at the time of admission showed bradycardia, with absent P waves, prolonged QRS complexes, and peak T waves. Her serum potassium concentration was found to be 7.5 mmol/L.**

   She has a left forearm AV fistula, and you plan to initiate her on emergency haemodialysis after administering calcium gluconate and insulin with dextrose.

   Which dialysate potassium concentration would you prescribe?

   A. 2 mmol/L
   B. 4 mmol/L
   C. 0 mmol/L
   D. 1 mmol/L
   E. 0.5 mmol/L

190. **A 62-year-old gentleman with ESRD secondary to hypertensive nephrosclerosis has been on haemodialysis for the past 2 years. He has no past history of ischaemic heart disease and is a lifelong non-smoker. He is concerned about his cardiac risk and seeks advice regarding treatment of his high cholesterol levels.**

> Investigations:
> serum cholesterol   6.2 mmol/L (<5.2)
> serum non-HDL-cholesterol   4.10 mmol/L (<3.36)
> serum HDL-cholesterol   1.05 mmol/L (>1.55)
> fasting serum triglycerides   2.3 mmol/L (0.45–2.30)

What would you advise the patient?

A. atorvastatin
B. PCSK9 inhibitor
C. ezetimibe
D. fenofibrate
E. statins are not indicated

191. **A 27-year-old lady on thrice-weekly haemodialysis was evaluated for amenorrhoea. Her pregnancy test was positive, and an ultrasound scan confirmed a viable fetus of 10 weeks' gestation. She has a residual urine output of 120 mL/day, and her BP is well controlled with nifedipine.**

Which modification to her dialysis prescription would improve fetal outcome?

A. 16-hour haemodialysis/week and maintain mid-week pre-dialysis urea <40 mmol/L
B. 18-hour haemodialysis/week and maintain mid-week pre-dialysis urea <50 mmol/L
C. 24-hour haemodialysis/week and maintain mid-week pre-dialysis urea <40 mmol/L
D. 24-hour haemodialysis/week and maintain mid-week pre-dialysis urea <35 mmol/L
E. 36-hour haemodialysis/week and maintain mid-week pre-dialysis urea <17.5 mmol/L

192. **A 66-year-old gentleman on thrice-weekly haemodialysis for the past 8 years, secondary to diabetic nephropathy, developed an intensely painful lesion on his back. This has been gradually increasing in size, along with ulceration.**

> Investigations:
> skin biopsy showed medial calcification, intimal proliferation of small vessels, along with fibrosis and areas of necrosis

Which one of the following treatments can definitively aid in the management of this condition?

A. continue current HD and initiate sodium thiosulfate
B. continue current HD and start broad-spectrum antibiotics
C. intensify HD and initiate sevelamer
D. intensify HD and initiate sodium thiosulfate
E. intensify HD and initiate vitamin D analogues

193. **A 45-year-old lady underwent a deceased donor renal transplant 2 weeks ago, with delayed graft function, and is on haemodialysis via a right internal jugular tunnelled dialysis catheter. She presents with a 3-day history of pain and redness in her right eye. A diagnosis of right eye endophthalmitis was made.**

> On clinical examination, the tunnel is healthy. Blood culture from the dialysis catheter hub and dialysis circuit culture grow *Candida albicans*.

What is the next most appropriate step in management?

A. intraluminal fluconazole and remove the dialysis catheter if no response
B. remove the dialysis catheter and exchange over a guidewire at the same site
C. remove the dialysis catheter and place a new catheter at a different site
D. systemic antifungal and exchange the dialysis catheter if no response
E. systemic antifungal and remove the dialysis catheter if no response

194. **A 60-year-old lady with hypertension and diabetes presented with uraemia and was started on haemodialysis. Twenty minutes into her first dialysis, she developed breathlessness, with itching and chest discomfort.**

> On examination, her BP was 90/62 mmHg and her heart rate was 124 beats/min. She had bilateral wheeze on chest auscultation. You suspect a dialyser reaction.

What is the most appropriate next step in management?

A. continue dialysis and administer IV steroids and antihistamines
B. continue dialysis and give a fluid bolus
C. continue dialysis and give salbutamol nebulizer
D. stop dialysis and give a fluid bolus
E. stop dialysis and do not return the blood back to the patient
F. stop dialysis and return the blood back to the patient

195. **A 62-year-old gentleman on haemodialysis for 2 years presented with a history of worsening exertional dyspnoea, fatigue, and pedal oedema for the past 6 months.**

> On examination, his BP was 130/88 mmHg and his JVP was 4 cm above the sternal angle. Cardiac examination revealed a systolic murmur in the left second intercostal space and his chest was clear. He had a large aneurysmal brachiocephalic arteriovenous fistula.
> You consider a diagnosis of high-output cardiac failure.

Which haemodynamic parameter would be consistent with high-output cardiac failure?

A. 10% decrease in EF after manually occluding the AVF
B. 10% increase in EF after manually occluding the AVF
C. mean pulmonary arterial pressure of 30 mmHg
D. Qa of >20% of cardiac output (Qa/CO) or access flow rate (Qa) of 1.5 L/min
E. Qa of 15% of cardiac output (Qa/CO) or access flow rate (Qa) of 1 mL/min

181. B. Echocardiography.

This patient has had a recent history of uraemic pericarditis that raises the possibility of the development of pericardial effusion. The disappearance of a pericardial friction rub in a patient with pericarditis could indicate resolution of pericarditis or the development of pericardial effusion. This patient who has presented with shock on a background of recent pericarditis requires urgent echocardiography to rule out cardiac tamponade. Cardiac tamponade is a life-threatening complication of pericarditis that has been reported to occur in approximately 10–20% of patients with uraemic/dialysis-associated pericarditis. Patients may present with hypotension, tachycardia, muffled heart sounds, and elevated JVP. Pulsus paradoxus, defined as an inspiratory decrease in systolic BP of >10 mmHg during normal breathing, is suggestive of tamponade and should lead to urgent further evaluation. Signs of tamponade on an echocardiogram include collapse of the right atrium and right ventricle during early diastole and increased variation in tricuspid and mitral valve blood flow velocity with respiration. The diagnosis of tamponade requires urgent pericardiocentesis to avoid cardiogenic shock and cardiac arrest. As the patient has cardiac tamponade and is already fluid-overloaded, administering a fluid challenge might worsen his condition. While starting haemodialysis, continuous renal replacement therapy or peritoneal dialysis are options for renal replacement therapy in a haemodynamically unstable patient. These modalities will not correct the primary cause of hypotension.

Dad T, Sarnak MJ. Pericarditis and pericardial effusions in end stage renal disease. Semin Dial. 2016;29(5):366–73.

Vijani P, Cherian SV, Gajjala Reddy N, *et al*. Acute decompensation after hemodialysis in a patient with pericardial effusion. Ann Am Thorac Soc. 2018;15(5):633–6.

182. E. Pericatheter fibrin sheath.

Catheter dysfunction can be classified as early or late. Causes of early catheter dysfunction include an improperly positioned catheter and a kinked catheter, as well as a catheter that is constricted by the exit site suture(s). If the catheter has been recently exchanged for a previously malfunctioning catheter, placement of the new catheter into a pre-existing fibrin sheath must also be considered as a possible cause of catheter malfunction. Late catheter dysfunction is defined as the inability to attain and maintain a blood flow rate sufficient to perform haemodialysis without significantly lengthening the haemodialysis treatment in a catheter that was previously functioning adequately. Late dysfunction of tunnelled catheters is usually due to a fibrin sheath which develops around the catheter and obstructs the arterial side holes, causing poor inflow in the arterial line, with excessive negative pressures generated during high pump speed required during dialysis. The presence of a fibrin sheath is diagnosed by contrast study. Thrombolytics may be beneficial, though the benefits are not sustained in the long term. Other available options include fibrin sheath stripping, internal snare, and over-the-wire catheter exchange with or without balloon disruption.

Daugirdas JT, Blake PG, Ing TS (eds). *Handbook of Dialysis*, 5th edition. Philadelphia, PA: Wolters Kluwer, 2015.

183. E. Strict universal precautions in the dialysis facility.

Isolation of HCV-infected patients (or patients awaiting HCV screening results) during haemodialysis sessions is defined as physical segregation from others for the express purpose of limiting direct or indirect transmission of HCV. Evidence of HCV transmission through internal pathways of the modern single-pass dialysis machine has not been demonstrated. Although contaminated external surfaces of dialysis machines may facilitate the spread of HCV, other surfaces within the dialysis treatment station are likely to have the same impact, which diminishes the purported value of using dedicated machines. In addition, using dedicated machines may trigger the perception that there is no longer a risk of nosocomial HCV transmission, and thus reduce the attention devoted by haemodialysis staff members to body fluid precautions. In most reported HCV outbreaks in haemodialysis centres, multiple lapses in infection control were identified and involved practices such as hand hygiene and glove use, injectable medication handling, and environmental surface disinfection.

Kidney Disease: Improving Global Outcomes (KDIGO) Hepatitis C Work Group. KDIGO 2018 Clinical Practice Guideline for the prevention, diagnosis, evaluation, and treatment of hepatitis C in chronic kidney disease. Kidney Int Suppl. 2018;8:91–165.

Fabrizi F, Messa P. Transmission of hepatitis C virus in dialysis units: a systematic review of reports on outbreaks. Int J Artif Organs. 2015;38:471–80.

184. E. Replace metoprolol with carvedilol.

Although there are no prospective studies to define intradialytic hypertension, the suggestion of an increase in mean arterial pressure of 15 mmHg above the starting mean arterial pressure is considered intradialytic hypertension. Similarly, the exact prevalence of intradialytic hypertension is not known but is reported to be between 5% and 15%. 'Dialysability' or clearance with haemodialysis of different antihypertensives should be considered when prescribing them. Beta-blockers, such as atenolol, acebutolol, and metoprolol, are extensively cleared with haemodialysis. Hence, use of a poorly dialysed beta-blocker, such as bisoprolol, propranolol, or carvedilol, would be favoured over that of metoprolol to prevent intradialytic hypertension; hence answer E is correct. Calcium channel blockers, as well as antihypertensives such as clonidine and prazosin, are generally not extensively cleared by haemodialysis. All ACE inhibitors, except for fosinopril, are extensively cleared by haemodialysis.

Chen J, Gul, A Sarnak MJ. Management of intradialytic hypertension: the ongoing challenge. Sem Dial. 2006;19:141–5.

Santos SF, Peixoto AJ, Perazella MA. How should we manage adverse intradialytic blood pressure changes? Adv Chronic Kidney Dis. 2012;19:158–65.

185. C. Reduce blood flow and dialysate flow.

Dialysis disequilibrium syndrome (DDS) is characterized by neurological signs and symptoms occurring during or shortly after an HD session. Clinical manifestations can include headache, nausea/vomiting, confusion, agitation, seizures, coma, and even death. Cerebral oedema may be seen on CT and MRI. DDS has been seen typically in patients with significantly elevated serum urea nitrogen levels undergoing their first dialysis treatment. Other risk factors include rapid reduction of blood urea nitrogen (BUN) levels, extremes of age, metabolic acidosis, hypo-/hypernatraemia, liver disease, and pre-existing neurological conditions.

The incidence of DDS is believed to have declined in recent decades due to changing practices such as starting dialysis with lower blood flow rates and at lower BUN levels. Prevention of DDS by reducing BUN levels by no more than 40% over a short period of time is crucial. Initiating HD using a low blood flow rateof 200 mL/min over 2 hours (or even less, depending on the patient's body habitus) is recommended. DDS has been reported in prevalent maintenance HD patients, so using a lower blood flow rate when such patients have significantly elevated BUN levels is also recommended. Another approach is to increase the osmolality in the blood or dialysate to reduce the degree of change in osmolality with dialysis. Use of a higher sodium dialysate has been reported to prevent symptoms of DDS. Other agents that have been used include mannitol, glucose, glycerol, and urea.

Greenberg KI, Choi MJ. Hemodialysis emergencies: core curriculum 2021. Am J Kidney Dis. 77(5):796–809.

Zepeda-Orozco D, Quigley R. Dialysis disequilibrium syndrome. Pediatr Nephrol. 2012;27(12): 2205–11.

186. B. Increase the frequency of haemodialysis and switch to a high-flux dialyser.

Dialysis-related amyloidosis (DRA) is characterized by tissue accumulation and deposition of amyloid fibrils consisting of beta-2 microglobulin in the bone, periarticular structures, and viscera of patients with CKD on long-standing haemodialysis of >8–10 years. Scapulohumeral periarthritis and carpal tunnel syndrome, as in the above case, can be manifestations of this disease. With use of high-flux dialysers, clearance of middle molecules, such as beta-2 microglobulin, can be improved. However, the endogenous production of beta-2 microglobulin far exceeds its removal, even with high-flux dialysers, along with 'rebound' in plasma levels of beta-2 microglobulin post-dialysis. Therefore, increasing dialysis treatment time, such as with daily nocturnal dialysis, as well as using a high-flux dialyser to improve convective clearance of beta-2 microglobulin, will help in this condition. Haemofiltration and haemodiafiltration do not provide a clear benefit, compared to that associated with biocompatible high-flux haemodialysis performed at high blood flow rates; hence, these modalities are not recommended at present solely for treatment of DRA. As the patient has no residual renal function, peritoneal dialysis is unlikely to be beneficial.

National Kidney Foundation. KDOQI Clinical Practice Guidelines for bone metabolism and disease in chronic kidney disease. Am J Kidney Dis. 2003;42(4 Suppl 3):S1–201.

Raj DS, Ouwendyk M, Francoeur R, Pierratos A. Beta(2)-microglobulin kinetics in nocturnal haemodialysis. Nephrol Dial Transplant. 2000;15(1):58–64.

Lerma, Edgar V, Weir, Matthew R. Beta2-microglobulin-associated amyloidosis of end-stage renal disease. In: WL Henrich, ed. *Principles and Practice of Dialysis*, 5th edition. Philadelphia, PA: Lippincott, Williams & Wilkins, 2016.

187. A. AVF angiography.

Recirculation is a common cause of inadequate dialysis delivery. Access recirculation is caused by low access blood flow rate. If access blood flow rate is less than the prescribed pump flow (typically 400–500 mL/min), backflow from the venous limb of the access is necessary to support the extracorporeal blood flow rate set by the blood pump. A major indication to measure recirculation in patients with either a fistula or a graft is that the delivered Kt/V is below target despite an adequate haemodialysis prescription. Recirculation is not the optimal method of surveillance for fistula stenosis and, if used as such, should only have a minor role. Significant recirculation tends to be a late marker of stenosis, which limits its utility.

Low access blood flow rate may be due to venous stenosis, intra-access stenosis, or arterial inflow stenosis. Recirculation does not result from placing needles too closely together as long as the access blood flow rate exceeds the machine blood flow rate. However, substantial recirculation (20% or more) is caused by reversed needle placement. Recirculation of 10% or more by a urea-based method should prompt further evaluation with fistulography, as it is more sensitive than a duplex ultrasound scan.

Basile C, Ruggieri G, Vernaglione L, et al. A comparison of methods for the measurement of hemodialysis access recirculation. J Nephrol. 2003;16:908.

Dinwiddie LC, Ball L, Brouwer D, et al. What nephrologists need to know about vascular access cannulation. Semin Dial. 2013;26:315.

Hemodialysis Adequacy 2006 Work Group. Clinical Practice Guidelines for hemodialysis adequacy, update 2006. Am J Kidney Dis. 2006;48(Suppl 1):S2.

188. B. Arm elevation test.

The pulse augmentation test is used to assess the direction of blood flow in AVF. The arm elevation test is a simple method to diagnose outflow vein stenosis. Under normal circumstances, when the fistula arm is raised above the level of the heart, the fistula will collapse. If an outflow stenosis is present, the area of the fistula distal to the stenosis will remain distended. This test works best with forearm AVFs and is not valid for AVGs. Patients can be taught to perform the arm elevation test as a way to self-monitor their AV accesses. Allen's test is used to evaluate the patency of the arteries in the hand prior to AVF surgery.

The sequential occlusion test is used to determine the presence of collateral veins. Similar to the pulse augmentation test, one hand is used to occlude the AV access outflow, while the other hand is used to palpate the thrill. The AV access is occluded progressively further down the venous outflow tract. If no collateral vein is present, no thrill will be felt. However, if a thrill is palpable despite occlusion of the AV access, that indicates the presence of a collateral vein below the point of occlusion. The Nicoladoni–Israel–Branham sign is a standard test of the haemodynamic significance of an AVF. A sudden occlusion of the AVF would be immediately followed by a decrease in the pulse rate and an increase in BP.

Abreo K, Amin BM, Abreo AP. Physical examination of the hemodialysis arteriovenous fistula to detect early dysfunction. J Vasc Access. 2019;20(1):7–11.

Coentrão L, Turmel-Rodrigues L. Monitoring dialysis arteriovenous fistulae: it's in our hands. J Vasc Access. 2013;14:209–15.

189. A. 2 mmol/L.

In a Dialysis Outcomes and Practice Patterns Study analysis, comparison between dialysate potassium concentrations of 3 mmol/L to 2 mmol/L showed no difference in the risk of all-cause mortality or an arrhythmia composite outcome (including sudden cardiac death and arrhythmia-related hospitalization), with minimal effect on pre-dialysis serum potassium concentrations. However, dialysate potassium concentrations of <2 mmol/L may lead to a rapid reduction in serum potassium concentrations and should be avoided, especially in patients with high pre-dialysis serum potassium concentrations. After HD, the ongoing shift of intracellular potassium to the extracellular space results in a rebound of serum potassium concentrations. A more rapid post-dialysis rebound of serum potassium concentrations may occur with a greater serum–dialysate potassium gradient. This fluctuation in serum potassium concentrations may increase intradialytic cell membrane polarization and potentially cause cardiac arrhythmia. The PORTEND study of patients on maintenance HD demonstrated a higher incidence of pre-dialysis hyperkalaemia after a long (2-day) interdialytic interval among patients on dialysate potassium concentrations of ≤2 mmol/L vs ≤3 mmol/L.

Zhang H, Douglas E Schaubel, John D Kalbfleisch, et al. Dialysis outcomes and analysis of practice patterns suggests the dialysis schedule affects day-of-week mortality. Kidney Int. 2012;81(11):1108–15.

Potassium and Cardiac Rhythm Trends in MaintENance HemoDialysis: a multicenter, prospective, observational study (PORTEND). ClinicalTrials.gov; NCT02609841. Accessible at https://clinicaltrials.gov/ct2/show/NCT02609841

190. E. Statins are not indicated.

Statins have shown a beneficial effect on all-cause and cardiovascular related mortality in non-dialysis CKD patients. However, their effect in HD patients is controversial. Initial studies have shown no CV benefit in HD patients. The 4D study (Deutsche Diabetes Dialyse Study) in 1255 HD patients with type 2 diabetes showed no benefit of atorvastatin (20 mg) during a mean follow-up of 4 years on any CV events. Although LDL-cholesterol levels were reduced, atorvastatin was associated with an increased risk of stroke.

Similarly, the AURORA (A Study to Evaluate the Use of Rosuvastatin in Subjects on Regular Dialysis) study on 2776 dialysis patients did not show any CV benefit during a 3.8-year follow-up. In the SHARP (Study of Heart and Renal Protection) study, use of simvastatin (20 mg) and ezetimibe (10 mg) for 4.9 years in 2527 HD and 496 PD patients did not have any effect on cardiovascular events.

The KDIGO guideline does not recommend the use of LDL-cholesterol level to assess the coronary risk in CKD patients. Based on the above large studies, initiation of statin therapy is not routinely recommended to prevent CV events in dialysis patients. However, if the patient is already on a statin, it should be continued. The 2014 Kidney Disease: Improving Global Outcomes Lipid Work Group suggests that statins should not be initiated in patients on dialysis, but they can be continued in patients already receiving them at the time of dialysis initiation.

Hou W, Lv J, Perkovic V, et al. Effect of statin therapy on cardiovascular and renal outcomes in patients with chronic kidney disease: a systematic review and meta-analysis. Eur Heart J. 2013;34:1807–17.

Kidney Disease: Improving Global Outcomes (KDIGO) Lipid Work Group. KDIGO Clinical Practice Guideline for lipid management in chronic kidney disease. Kidney Int Suppl. 2013;3:259–305.

191. E. 36-hour haemodialysis/week and maintain mid-week pre-dialysis urea <17.5 mmol/L.

There is a strong association between increased dialysis dose and improved fertility and pregnancy outcomes. Pregnant women who receive longer dialysis have higher conception rates, as well as higher live birth rates and heavier babies at birth. Maternal urea levels were much lower in pregnancies with successful outcomes, aiming for a pre-dialysis urea level of <12.5 mmol/L. Frequent dialysis also allows higher protein intake and reduces the risk of intradialytic hypotension, which can be detrimental to fetal development.

Hladunewich MA, Hou S, Odutayo A, et al. Intensive hemodialysis associates with improved pregnancy outcomes: a Canadian and United States cohort comparison. J Am Soc Nephrol. 2014;25:1103–9.

Wiles K, Chappell L, Clark K, et al. Clinical practice guideline on pregnancy and renal disease. BMC Nephrol. 2019;20:401.

Williams D. Pregnancy with pre-existing kidney disease. In: J Feehally, J Floege, RJ Johnson, eds. *Comprehensive Clinical Nephrology*, 3rd edition. Philadelphia, PA: Mosby, 2007; pp. 485–504.

192. D. Intensify HD and initiate sodium thiosulfate.

This patient has calciphylaxis (calcific uraemic arteriolopathy) of his lower back. Calcific uraemic arteriolopathy, or calciphylaxis, is an uncommon, but potentially devastating, complication of abnormal mineral metabolism. Calciphylaxis is characterized by painful skin ulceration with necrosis, and medial calcification. It occurs more frequently in chronic HD patients than in non-dialysis patients. The incidence varies from <1% to 4%. Traditional risk factors include secondary hyperparathyroidism, hypercalcaemia, hyperphosphataemia, calcium-based phosphate binders, obesity, diabetes, protein C deficiency, female sex, warfarin use, and low albumin. The mortality rate at 1 year varies between 45% and 55%. There is no definitive treatment. Although no prospective studies are available regarding treatment efficacy, multi-interventional treatment is recommended, which includes avoidance of calcium-based binder, vitamin D, and warfarin therapy. Institution of aggressive wound management and antibiotic use, intensification of HD (4-hour daily for 7 days, followed by 5–6 times weekly), and long-term sodium thiosulfate 12.5–25 g IV thrice weekly with oxygen therapy via a face mask have proven to benefit patients with calciphylaxis. A recent Australian retrospective study showed that sodium thiosulfate infusion (25 g thrice weekly) in HD patients for a median of 96 days resulted in complete remission in 14 of 27 (52%) patients. Besides chelating calcium, sodium thiosulfate may have other effects in improving calciphylaxis. Thus, option D is correct. Other therapeutic modalities include bisphosphonates, cinacalcet, and corticosteroids to improve inflammation, surgery to the wound, and hyperbaric oxygen.

Baldwin C, Farah M, Leung M, et al. Multi-intervention management of calciphylaxis: a report of 7 cases. Am J Kidney Dis. 2011;58:988–91.

Ross EA. Evolution of treatment strategies for calciphylaxis. Am J Nephrol. 2011;34:460–7.

Vedvyas C, Winterfield LS, Vleugels RA. Calciphylaxis: a systematic review of existing and emerging therapies. J Am Acad Dermatol. 2012;67:e253–60.

193. C. Remove the dialysis catheter and place a new catheter at a different site.

Several situations necessitate immediate CVC removal, with delayed CVC placement:

1. clinically and haemodynamically unstable patients
2. persistent fever 48–72 hours after initiation of systemic antibiotics
3. persistent bacteraemia 48–72 hours after initiating antibiotics
4. metastatic complications, including suppurative thrombophlebitis and endocarditis
5. infections due to *Staphylococcus aureus*, *Pseudomonas aeruginosa*, fungi, or mycobacteria
6. presence of a tunnel site infection.

In this patient with *Candida* fungaemia, with metastatic fungal endophthalmitis, the best option would be to remove the CVC, replace it at a new site, and treat with a prolonged course of antifungals.

Lok CE, Huber TS, Lee T, et al.; KDOQI Vascular Access Guideline Work Group. KDOQI Clinical Practice Guideline for vascular access: 2019 update. Am J Kidney Dis. 2020;75(4 Suppl 2):S1–164.

194. E. Stop dialysis and do not return the blood back to the patient.

Dialyser reactions are hypersensitivity reactions to the membrane or the products used to sterilize the membrane. The reactions were fairly common previously but rarely seen nowadays due to increased use of biocompatible membranes and reduced use of ethylene oxide sterilization. Dialyser reactions have been described as type A or type B. Type A reactions occur early in treatment, usually within the first 20–30 minutes. They typically occur during the first treatment but can occur after multiple treatments. Signs and symptoms may include itching, laryngeal oedema, bronchospasm, dyspnoea, chest pain, vomiting, hypoxia, hypotension, and cardiac arrest. Management of a severe reaction includes stopping dialysis without returning blood from the extracorporeal circuit back into the patient. In addition, patients can be given steroids, nebulizers, and antihistamines as required.

Type B reactions occur later in treatment and tend to be less severe. Symptoms may include chest and back pain, nausea, and vomiting. Dialysis can be continued if symptoms are mild.

Greenberg KI, Choi MJ. Hemodialysis emergencies: core curriculum 2021. Am J Kidney Dis. 77(5):796–809.

Saha M, Allon M. Diagnosis, treatment, and prevention of hemodialysis emergencies. Clin J Am Soc Nephrol. 2017;12(2):357–69.

195. D. Qa of >20% of cardiac output (Qa/CO) or access flow rate (Qa) of 1.5 L/min.

Cardinal symptoms of congestive cardiac failure, such as dyspnoea and fatigue, can be exacerbated by AV access, as they can lead to high-output failure. High flow rates through an AV access can lead to a number of detrimental effects, which include high-output congestive heart failure, pulmonary hypertension (generally over 50 mmHg in such cases), central venous stenosis, venous hypertension, aneurysmal degeneration of the AVF, and AV access-related hand ischaemia. The exact threshold to define high-flow access has not been universally accepted, although an AV access flow rate (Qa) of 1–1.5 L/min or a Qa of >20% of the cardiac output (Qa/CO) is considered high enough.

Basile *et al.* reported that Qa values of >2.0 L/min were associated with the occurrence of high-output cardiac failure, with a sensitivity of 89% and a specificity of 100%, whereas a Qa/CO of ≤20% had a sensitivity of 100% and a specificity of 75%. AV access flow rates can be reduced by using a variety of flow-reducing therapies or banding. In patients with high-flow AVFs (Qa >2.0 L/min), occlusion of the AVF leads to a markedly reduced cardiac index. Resolution of symptoms and intracardiac pressures after occlusion/closure is the sine qua non of diagnosis.

Basile C, Lomonte C, Vernaglione L, et al. The relationship between the flow of arteriovenous fistula and cardiac output in haemodialysis patients. Nephrol Dial Transplant. 2008;23:282–7.

Lok CE, Huber TS, Lee T, et al.; KDOQI Vascular Access Guideline Work Group. KDOQI Clinical Practice Guideline for vascular access: 2019 update. Am J Kidney Dis. 2020;75(4 Suppl 2):S1–164.

Take-Home Messages

1. Dialysability of antihypertensives should be taken into account when prescribing antihypertensives for HD patients.
2. Dialysis disequilibrium is a rare complication of HD and can be avoided by doing a shorter dialysis session with lower blood flow rate and dialysate flow rate.
3. Recirculation is a common cause of inadequate dialysis.
4. More frequent dialysis is associated with reduced maternal and perinatal morbidity in pregnant dialysis patients.
5. Calciphylaxis is an uncommon, but serious, complication in dialysis patients and can be treated with frequent HD and sodium thiosulfate.
6. Dialyser reactions are rare with biocompatible membranes.
7. Though AVFs have the lowest complication rate, they can be rarely associated with high-output heart failure.
8. A positive sodium gradient during HD can lead to high intra-dialytic weight gain which is associated with increased cardiovascular morbidity and mortality.
9. Water used for HD should comply with established quality standards and be checked periodically for microbial and chemical contamination.
10. Nocturnal and short daily HD may be associated with improved patient survival, compared to conventional in-centre HD.

chapter 12

RENAL TRANSPLANTATION

QUESTIONS

196. A 72-year-old man underwent a deceased donor renal transplant 3 months ago for diabetic nephropathy. Routine post-transplant virology screening showed BK viraemia of 15,000 copies/mL. His graft function was stable. Current medications comprised tacrolimus 3 mg twice a day, mycophenolate sodium 720 mg twice a day, and prednisolone 5 mg daily.

Investigations:	
serum creatinine	72 µmol/L (60–90)
serum urea	5.0 mmol/L (2.5–7)
serum sodium	139 mmol/L (135–145)
serum potassium	4.2 mmol/L (3.5–5.0)
blood tacrolimus (trough)	7 nmol/L (8.0–12.0)

What is the most appropriate next step?

A. cidofovir

B. ciprofloxacin

C. increase tacrolimus

D. leflunomide

E. reduce mycophenolate sodium

Best of Five MCQs for the European Specialty Examination in Nephrology. Shafi Malik, Oxford University Press.
 DOI: 10.1093/oso/9780192844163.003.0023

197. **A 56-year-old Caucasian lady was seen in the live donor assessment clinic and wished to donate a kidney to her husband who was on dialysis. Other than hypertension, for which she was on amlodipine, there was no other significant past history. There was no family history of renal disease.**

    On examination, her BP was 135/80 mmHg and her BMI was 30 kg/m². All peripheral pulses were palpable.

    Investigations:
    serum creatinine   60 µmol/L (60–90)
    eGFR   95 mL/min (60–90)
    urine protein:creatinine ratio 10 mg/mmol (<30)
    ultrasound scan of kidneys   normal-sized kidneys with normal appearances

    What would be her lifetime risk of ESRD if she were to donate?

    A. 0.5–1%
    B. 5–10%
    C. 10–15%
    D. 25–30%
    E. 3–4%

198. **A 36-year-old man was seen in the transplant outpatient clinic. He had undergone a deceased donor renal transplant 10 days ago, with basiliximab induction. Maintenance immunosuppression included tacrolimus, mycophenolate mofetil, and prednisolone. The cause of his end-stage renal disease was membranous nephropathy. HLA mismatch was 2-2-2.**

    On examination, the patient was euvolaemic and his BP was 145/90 mmHg.

    Investigations:
    serum creatinine   120 µmol/L (60–90)
    eGFR   66 mL/min (60–90)

    He was reviewed a week later and below are investigations at this visit.

    serum creatinine   200 µmol/L (60–90)
    eGFR   36 mL/min (60–90)
    urine protein:creatinine ratio 10 mg/mmol (<30)
    blood tacrolimus (trough)   3.2 nmol/L (8.0–12.0)
    transplant biopsy   (see Fig)

    What is the next best step in management?

    A. alemtuzumab
    B. increase tacrolimus
    C. IVIg
    D. pulsed methylprednisolone
    E. repeat transplant biopsy

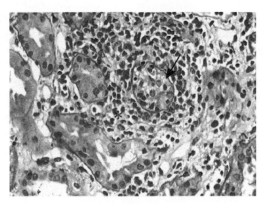

Reproduced with permission from Torpey, Nicholas and others (eds), *Renal Transplantation*, Oxford Specialist Handbooks (Oxford, 2010; online edn, Oxford Academic, 1 Oct 2011), https://doi.org/10.1093/med/9780199215669.001.1, accessed 11 Nov 2022.

199. **A 56-year-old gentleman with end-stage renal disease due to type 2 diabetes was seen in the transplant assessment clinic. He was referred for transplant workup. He has been experiencing hypoglycaemic unawareness. Other than hypertension, there was no other significant past history. He was on a total of 50 units of insulin per day. His BMI was 29 kg/m². Workup investigations were satisfactory.**

    What would you advise the patient?

    A. islet cell transplant

    B. kidney transplant

    C. not suitable for transplantation

    D. pancreas alone transplant

    E. simultaneous pancreas–kidney transplant

200. **A 62-year-old lady was seen in the transplant assessment clinic. She is currently pre-dialysis, and the cause of her end-stage renal disease is renovascular disease. She had a past history of melanoma *in situ* on her back diagnosed 2 years ago, which was completely excised, and she received no further treatment. Workup investigations were satisfactory.**

    What would be the next best step?

    A. list for renal transplant

    B. not suitable for transplantation

    C. refer to dermatology

    D. wait for three more years

    E. wait for two more years

201. **A 20-year-old lady was seen in the renal outpatient clinic. She underwent a live donor renal transplant a month ago. She was otherwise well and has no significant past history. She enquires about inactivated COVID-19 vaccination.**

Investigations:

serum creatinine	89 µmol/L (60–110)
white cell count	5.01×10^9/L (4.0–11.0)
platelet count	158×10^9/L (150–400)

What should be your advice?

A. can have it now

B. vaccination not indicated

C. vaccination is contraindicated

D. wait for two more months

E. wait for a year

202. **A 59-year-old man on home haemodialysis was seen in the transplant assessment clinic. He was found to be fit for transplant listing. His wife has been worked up as a live donor. The recipient's blood group is O, and the donor's blood group is A2.**

Investigations:

flow crossmatch	negative
A2 titre	1:8

What would be the next best management step?

A. directed live donor transplant

B. IVIg

C. paired exchange scheme

D. plasma exchange

E. rituximab

203. **A 69-year-old man was seen in the transplant outpatient clinic. He underwent a live donor transplant 20 years ago, which is currently failing. He was short of breath at rest and had lower limb oedema. There is a plan to start him on haemodialysis on the following day via a functioning AV fistula. He continues to pass some urine, and current medications include mycophenolate, tacrolimus, and prednisolone.**

What would be the most appropriate next step?

A. stop mycophenolate

B. stop mycophenolate and prednisolone

C. stop mycophenolate and tacrolimus

D. stop prednisolone

E. stop tacrolimus

204. **A 26-year-old woman is worked up as an altruistic live donor. She has recently seen an urgent Facebook campaign for a 9-year-old child who is on dialysis, and now wishes to donate directly to this child. Workup is complete, and the patient is fit to donate.**

What would be your advice?

A. can donate

B. cannot donate

C. it is illegal

D. paired exchange scheme

E. second opinion

205. **A 35-year-old man is referred urgently by his GP to the transplant clinic with lower abdominal pain and haematuria for the past 3 days. He had undergone a renal transplant 15 years ago, which is now failing. Mycophenolate was stopped recently. He also admits to being non-compliant with other medications.**

On examination, his temperature was 37.7°C and his BP was 120/70 mmHg. Abdominal examination showed graft tenderness.

Investigations:

serum urea	36 mmol/L (2.5–7.0)
serum creatinine	480 µmol/L (60–110)
serum sodium	137 mmol/L (137–144)
serum potassium	6.0 mmol/L (3.5–4.9)
white cell count	7.0 × 10⁹/L (4.0–11.0)

What is the next best management step?

A. graft nephrectomy

B. IV methylprednisolone

C. meropenem

D. oral prednisolone

E. restart mycophenolate

206. **A 40-year-old man was seen in the transplant clinic. He had undergone a renal transplant 12 months ago. He was on prednisolone, azathioprine, and tacrolimus for maintenance immunosuppression.**

On examination, he was euvolaemic and his BP was 128/70 mmHg.

Investigations:

serum creatinine	86 µmol/L (60–110)
haemoglobin	190 g/L (130–180)
white cell count	6600 × 10⁹/L (4.0–11.0)
platelet count	170,000 × 10⁹/L (150–400)
CT scan of thorax and abdomen	normal

What is the most appropriate next step?

A. amlodipine
B. aspirin
C. atorvastatin
D. clopidogrel
E. ramipril

207. **A 50-year-old woman presents to the transplant clinic with a 2-day history of flu-like symptoms. She had undergone a renal transplant 2 months ago and is currently on mycophenolate, tacrolimus, and prednisolone maintenance.**

On examination, her temperature was 37.5°C and her BP was 120/60 mmHg. Her chest was clear.

Investigations:

serum creatinine	96 µmol/L (60–110)
serum urea	4.8 mmol/L (2.5–7.0)
white cell count	2.4 × 10⁹/L (4.0–11.0)
platelet count	110 × 10⁹/L (150–400)

Which is the most appropriate treatment?

A. cidofovir
B. ganciclovir
C. IVIg
D. valaciclovir
E. valganciclovir

208. **A 35-year-old man presented to the transplant clinic 2 weeks after his DCD renal transplant. The cause of ESRD was Alport syndrome.**

Urinalysis showed blood 3+ and protein 3+.

Investigations:
serum creatinine   110 µmol/L (60–110)

He returned a week later and investigations at this visit were:

serum creatinine   240 µmol/L (60–110)
blood tacrolimus (trough)   9.2 nmol/L (8.0–12.0)
ultrasound scan of renal transplant   good perfusion, no collection or hydronephrosis

Which of the following is the most likely cause of graft dysfunction?

A. acute rejection
B. anti-GBM disease
C. CNI toxicity
D. *de novo* FSGS
E. recurrence of Alport syndrome

209. **A 60-year-old man was referred by his GP to the renal clinic for investigation of weight loss. He had undergone a renal transplant 10 years ago. He was on belatacept and prednisolone as maintenance immunosuppression.**

Investigations:
serum creatinine   96 µmol/L (60–110)
FDG-PET scan   multiple lymphadenopathies in the retroperitoneum and mediastinum
Epstein-Barr virus viral load   100,000 copies/mL (lower detection limit 100)
lymph node biopsy   awaited

What would be the most appropriate treatment for this condition?

A. leflunomide
B. prednisolone
C. R-CHOP
D. reduce immunosuppression
E. rituximab

210. A 60-year-old man presented to the renal clinic for routine review. He had a renal transplant 2 years ago. He was recently treated for a lower respiratory tract infection with antibiotics by the GP. current medications were prednisolone, mycophenolate, and tacrolimus.

Investigations:

serum creatinine	90 µmol/L (60–110)
serum urea	3.4 mmol/L (2.5–7.0)
blood tacrolimus (trough)	15 nmol/L (8.0–12.0)

Which of the following can explain the tacrolimus level?

A. amoxicillin–clavulanate

B. azithromycin

C. co-trimoxazole

D. doxycycline

E. levofloxacin

211. A 70-year-old man was seen in the renal clinic. He had a renal transplant 10 years ago. Current medications were metformin, prednisolone, ciclosporin, and amlodipine.

Investigations:

serum creatinine	90 µmol/L (60–110)
urine protein:creatinine ratio	600 mg/mmol (<30)
free light chain	kappa 110 mg/L; lambda 210 mg/L
protein electrophoresis	no M spike
haemoglobin A1c	54 mmol/mol (20–42)
renal biopsy	(see Fig)

What is the most likely diagnosis?

A. amyloidosis

B. diabetic nephropathy

C. fibrillary glomerulopathy

D. immunotactoid glomerulopathy

E. membranous nephropathy

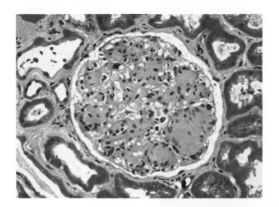

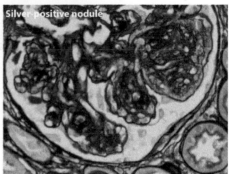

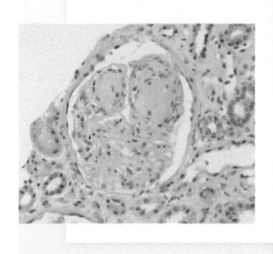

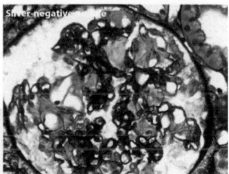

212. **A 35-year-old man was seen in the transplant clinic for follow-up of his ABO-incompatible renal transplant done 4 weeks ago. Blood types were donor A1-positive to recipient O-positive. He had a donor-specific antibody for HLA-DQ5, with an MFI of 500.**

Investigations:

serum creatinine	80 µmol/L (60–110)
urine albumin:creatinine ratio	30 mg/mmol (<2.5)

A week later:

serum creatinine	160 µmol/L (60–110)
blood tacrolimus (trough)	12.4 nmol/L (8.0–12.0)
anti-A titre	1:16 K

renal transplant biopsy (see Fig)

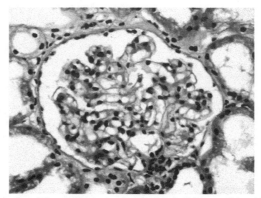

Reproduced with permission from Winearls, Christopher G. and others (ed.), 'The renal biopsy', in Neil N. Turner and others (eds), *Oxford Textbook of Clinical Nephrology*: Three-Volume Pack, 4 edn (Oxford, 2015; online edn, Oxford Academic, 1 June 2019), https://doi.org/10.1093/med/9780199592548.003.0018_update_001, accessed 6 Dec 2022.

What is the most likely cause of graft dysfunction?

A. acute tubular necrosis

B. antibody-mediated rejection

C. calcineurin inhibitor toxicity

D. cellular rejection

E. polyoma virus nephropathy

213. **A 50-year-old woman with a functioning renal transplant presented with accelerated hypertension and pulmonary oedema. She was started on ramipril 2 weeks ago, as her BP was consistently around 170/100 mmHg.**

    On examination, her BP was 180/110 mmHg, and she had lower limb oedema and fine crepitations in both lung bases.

    Investigations:
    serum creatinine   190 µmol/L (60–110)
    serum urea   5.3 mmol/L (2.5–7.0)
    serum potassium   6.2 mmol/L (3.5–4.9)

    Which investigation is most likely to confirm the diagnosis?

    A. CT angiography
    B. Doppler ultrasound
    C. transthoracic echocardiography
    D. plasma renin and aldosterone levels
    E. renal biopsy

214. **A 45-year-old woman is seen in the outpatient clinic. She had undergone a renal transplant 10 years ago for FSGS. She was on ciclosporin and prednisolone. She complained of worsening lower limb oedema and is known to have a *de novo* DSA DQ5 MFI of 12,000.**

    Investigations:
    serum creatinine   240 µmol/L (60–110)
    serum creatinine 6 months ago   190 µmol/L (60–110)
    serum albumin   32 g/L (37–49)
    urine protein:creatinine ratio   400 mg/mmol (<30)

    Transplant biopsy showed double contouring of the GBM.

    What is the likely cause of graft dysfunction?

    A. acute rejection
    B. *de novo* MPGN
    C. interstitial fibrosis and tubular atrophy
    D. recurrent FSGS
    E. transplant glomerulopathy

215. **A 35-year-old man was admitted with graft dysfunction. He underwent a renal transplant 3 months ago for atypical haemolytic uraemic syndrome due to a membrane cofactor protein mutation. Induction immunosuppression included basiliximab. Current maintenance immunosuppression included prednisolone, tacrolimus, and sirolimus. Baseline creatinine level was 92 mmol/L.**

Investigations:

serum creatinine	300 µmol/L (60–110)
haemoglobin	80 g/L (130–180)
platelet count	100,000 × 10^9/L (150–400)
renal transplant biopsy	thrombotic microangiopathy and negative C4d

Which of the following can explain the graft dysfunction?

A. antibody-mediated rejection

B. hypertension

C. passenger lymphocyte syndrome

D. recurrence of aHUS

E. sirolimus

196. E. Reduce mycophenolate sodium.

BK viraemia affects 10–30% of renal transplants and typically starts appearing from 2 months post-transplant. The mainstay of treatment is reduction of immunosuppression. Anti-proliferatives, such as mycophenolate mofetil or azathioprine, are reduced by 50% as the first step (aiming for a total daily dose of <1 g or its equivalent). If after aggressive reduction of immunosuppression, BK viraemia persists, the next step would be to add adjunctive therapy such as leflunomide or cidofovir. There is no role for ciprofloxacin in treatment of BK viraemia.

Fishman JA. Infection in organ transplantation. Am J Transplant. 2017;4:856–79.

Hirsch HH, Randhawa P; AST Infectious Diseases Community of Practice. BK polyomavirus in solid organ transplantation. Am J Transplant. 2013;13(Suppl 4):179–88.

197. A. 0.5–1%.

Long-term follow-up cohort studies have shown a very small absolute increase in the lifetime risk of ESRD. The risk of ESRD is higher in younger donors, those with a family history of renal disease, and Afro-Caribbeans. The risk is estimated to be around 0.5% for this donor. The effect of well-controlled hypertension by non-pharmacological methods or one to two antihypertensive drugs on long-term outcome is not clear. Evidence of end-organ damage due to hypertension is a contraindication to donation. A BMI of 25–30 kg/m^2 in an otherwise healthy individual would be considered low risk. Risk calculators have now been developed to estimate risk and inform patients of the lifetime risk of ESRD (available from: http://www.trans plantmodels.com).

British Transplantation Society (2018). Guidelines for living donor kidney transplantation, 4th edition. https://bts.org.uk/guidelines-standards/

198. D. Pulsed methylprednisolone.

Biopsy shows tubulitis consistent with T cell-mediated rejection. In the 3C study, 17% of basiliximab-treated patients had acute rejection, compared to 7% in the alemtuzumab arm. There is a higher risk of delayed graft function in deceased donor transplants, which is a risk factor for acute rejection. Initial treatment would be with pulsed methylprednisolone. Steroid-resistant rejection may need treatment with T cell-depleting therapy such as alemtuzumab or ATG. Antibody-mediated rejection can be treated with IVIg.

Cooper JE. Evaluation and treatment of acute rejection in kidney allografts. Clin J Am Soc Nephrol. 2020;15(3):430–8.

199. E. Simultaneous pancreas–kidney transplant.

Simultaneous pancreas–kidney (SPK) transplants for type 2 diabetes have comparable graft and patient outcomes to transplants for type 1 diabetes. However, there are strict criteria for SPK transplants. Eligibility criteria for type 2 diabetic patients are insulin-dependent diabetes, fasting C-peptide <2.0 ng/mL, BMI ≤30 kg/m², and insulin requirements generally <75 U/day. SPK transplant would offer the best outcome, compared to other options.

British Transplantation Society (2019). UK guidelines on pancreas and islet transplantation. Available from: https://bts.org.uk/guidelines-standards/

200. A. List for renal transplant.

Immunosuppression is a risk factor for cancer progression. Transplant recipients with a past history of malignancy need to wait for a specified time free of disease prior to being considered for solid organ transplant. Waiting time varies by type of cancer and stage. However, melanoma *in situ* is not an invasive cancer, as long as the lesion has been excised completely. No waiting time is required, given the morbidity and mortality on dialysis. Proceeding with a transplant in such patients would not be high risk.

Lim WH, Au E, Krishnan A, et al. Assessment of kidney transplant suitability for patients with prior cancers: is it time for a rethink? Transpl Int. 2019;32(12):1223–40.

Zwald FO, Christenson LJ, Billingsley EM, et al.; Melanoma Working Group of The International Transplant Skin Cancer Collaborative and Skin Care in Organ Transplant Patients, Europe. Melanoma in solid organ transplant recipients. Am J Transplant. 2010;10(5):1297–304.

201. D. Wait for two more months.

Immunosuppressed patients are at higher risk of COVID-19. However, response to COVID-19 vaccination in transplant recipients has been variable. There is likely to be poor response to vaccination if given early post-transplant when immunosuppression doses would be high. A minimum period of 3 months post-transplant is recommended.

British Transplantation Society. Vaccination against COVID-19: FAQs for clinicians and patients. Available from: https://bts.org.uk/information-resources/covid-19-information/

202. A. Directed live donor transplant.

Live donor transplant offers better graft and patient outcomes, compared to deceased donor transplants. However, in those with an immunologically incompatible donor or those with age or size mismatch, enrolling donor–recipient pairs in the paired exchange scheme would offer them the potential of finding a better-suited donor. A2 to O would be low immunological risk, as ABO subgroup A2 expresses lower levels of A antigen on the cell surface and is less immunogenic towards anti-A immunoglobulin present in blood group O or B recipients. Directed transplant without any additional immunosuppression would be acceptable.

Azzi Y, Nair G, Loarte-Campos P, et al. A safe anti-A2 titer for a successful A2 incompatible kidney transplantation: a single-center experience and review of the literature. Transplant Direct. 2021;7(2):e662.

203. A. Stop mycophenolate.

Preparation of patients with a failing graft for renal replacement therapy is important, paying attention to education, access, renal bone disease, renal anaemia management, and workup for repeat transplantation if suitable. When patients return to dialysis following graft failure, anti-proliferatives, such as mycophenolate or azathioprine, are generally stopped due to a higher risk of infection and malignancy related to these drugs. Dialysis is also an immunocompromised state. If patients have urine output, it would be beneficial to maintain residual renal function for better survival. Tacrolimus can be continued in order for patients to maintain this with low target drug levels. In patients who are likely to be retransplanted within the next year, it would not be unreasonable to continue mycophenolate, in addition to tacrolimus and prednisolone, to reduce sensitization. Prednisolone should not be stopped suddenly.

Andrews PA; Standards Committee of the British Transplantation Society. Summary of the British Transplantation Society guidelines for management of the failing kidney transplant. Transplantation. 2014;98(11):1130–3.

204. A. Can donate.

Altruistic donors are encouraged to be enrolled in the paired exchange scheme as non-directed donors in order to trigger additional transplants. However, it would not be illegal or unacceptable for altruistic donors to donate to a recipient with no genetic or emotional relationship. It is not unusual for recipients to post the need for a donor on social media. It would be possible to donate to a recipient with whom the donor has come into contact via social media, as long as the recipient did not pay for advertising. Directed altruistic donor (DAD) referrals that arise from paid advertising or via websites where potential transplant recipients pay a fee to register their need for an organ transplant will not be accepted for living donor assessment. This is due to a lack of clarity in the motivation for donation in these cases and the associated difficulty of ruling out coercion and/or reward. Provided that payment has not been made for advertising, DAD referrals that arise from advertising and/or awareness campaigns via social networking sites or media stories will be considered for living donor assessment.

British Transplantation Society (2015). Directed altruistic organ donation. https://bts.org.uk/guidelines-standards/operational-guidelines/

British Transplantation Society (2018). Guidelines for living donor kidney transplantation, 4th edition. https://bts.org.uk/guidelines-standards/

205. B. IV methylprednisolone.

This is graft intolerance syndrome, a condition in which the patient is unable to tolerate an allograft after loss of function. Symptoms include fever, flu-like symptoms, malaise, haematuria, localized pain, renal transplant enlargement, and refractory anaemia with elevated CRP. Immunosuppression withdrawal can either worsen or cause chronic rejection. Graft nephrectomy is indicated, but the first-line treatment would be augmentation of immunosuppression with pulsed methylprednisolone. Graft nephrectomy is also indicated when symptoms are refractory to steroid treatment. In some case series, graft nephrectomy has led to increased sensitization as the graft in some cases acts as a sponge for HLA antibodies.

Davis S, Mohan S. Managing patients with failing kidney allograft. Clin J Am Soc Nephrol. 2022;17(3):444–51.

206. E. Ramipril.

Post-transplant erythrocytosis (PTE) is persistently elevated haemoglobin, not associated with leukocytosis or thrombocytosis. It occurs in 8–15% of kidney transplant recipients. Risk factors include male sex, rejection-free course, preserved GFR, hypertension, diuretic use, and long dialysis vintage. It is commonly seen 8–24 months post-transplant. It is important to rule out malignancy, COPD, obstructive sleep apnoea and transplant renal artery stenosis, before a diagnosis of PTE is made. Treatment of PTE includes ACEi/ARBs and venesection. Theophylline is used as a second-line agent. Aspirin is used as prophylaxis to prevent transplant renal vein thrombosis.

Alzoubi B, Kharel A, Machhi R, et al. Post-transplant erythrocytosis after kidney transplantation: a review. World J Transplant. 2021;11(6):220–30.

207. E. Valganciclovir.

This is CMV viral syndrome, which is the commonest presentation of CMV reactivation or primary infection. Mild–moderate disease can be treated with treatment-dose oral valganciclovir (double prophylaxis dose), whereas CMV disease needs treatment with IV ganciclovir or when gastrointestinal absorption may be poor. In life-threatening cases, CMV-specific IVIg can be used. Valaciclovir can be used for CMV prophylaxis. However, the risk of acute rejection is higher with its use. British Transplant Society guidelines recommend CMV prophylaxis with valganciclovir in CMV D+R− renal transplants. The duration of valganciclovir prophylaxis should be at least 100 days.

British Transplantation Society (2015). The prevention and management of CMV disease after solid organ transplantation, 3rd edition. https://bts.org.uk/uk-guideline-on-prevention-and-management-of-cytomegalovirus-cmv-infection-and-disease-following-solid-organ-transplantation/

Razonable RR, Humar A. Cytomegalovirus in solid organ transplant recipients: guidelines of the American Society of Transplantation Infectious Diseases Community of Practice. Clin Transplant. 2019;33(9):e13512.

Reischig T, Kacer M, Jindra P, et al. Randomized trial of valganciclovir versus valacyclovir prophylaxis for prevention of cytomegalovirus in renal transplantation. Clin J Am Soc Nephrol. 2015;10(2):294–304.

208. B. Anti-GBM disease.

Mutations in alpha chains of type IV collagen result in Alport syndrome. These patients are deficient in type IV collagen in the GBM, which results in progressive renal dysfunction leading to ESRD. Following renal transplantation, patients with Alport syndrome may develop anti-GBM antibodies as an alloimmune response to the neo-antigens contained in 'normal' $\alpha3$, $\alpha4$, or $\alpha5$ chains in the kidney allograft. Commercially available anti-GBM assays, which are optimized to detect reactivity to the $\alpha3(IV)NC1$ antigen, may fail to detect circulating antibodies in this setting. Anti-GBM antibodies may be detected in 5–10% of Alport syndrome patients after transplantation, although the development of overt glomerulonephritis in the allograft is less frequent. When GN develops, however, it usually occurs early and carries a high risk of graft loss.

Alport syndrome does not recur in renal allografts. The presence of blood and protein on a background of these findings is suggestive of glomerulonephritis (see Table 12.1).

Table 12.1 Recurrence Rate of Glomerular Diseases Post Renal Transplant

	Clinical recurrence rate (%)*	Graft loss after 5–10 years (%)*
IgA nephropathy	10–25 (>50 histological)	2–16
FSGS	20–40**	10–20
Immune complex-mediated MPGN	30–66	10–50
Complement-mediated MPGN	70–90	10–50
HUS	Classical 1 Atypical 20 Familial 80	Uncommon 55–100 Up to 100
Membranous nephropathy	5–30	5–20
Anti-GBM disease	Exceptional	Exceptional
ANCA-associated vasculitis	20	30
Lupus nephritis	5–30	<10

Adapted with permission from Barratt, Jonathan and others (eds), 'Renal transplantation', in Jonathan Barratt and others (eds), *Oxford Desk Reference Nephrology*, 2 edn (Oxford, 2021; online edn, Oxford Academic, 1 June 2021), https://doi.org/10.1093/med/9780198777182.003.0015

McAdoo SP, Pusey CD. Anti-glomerular basement membrane disease. Clin J Am Soc Nephrol. 2017;12(7):1162–72.

209. C. R-CHOP.

EBV seronegativity and induction therapy play a major role in the development of Post Transplant Lymphoproliferative Disease (PTLD). Early PTLD (within a year post-transplant) is usually EBV-driven; late PTLD may or may not be EBV-driven. EBV-negative PTLD is considered a lymphoma occurring coincidentally in a transplant patient. Tumour EBV status is not prognostic or predictive with respect to treatment response in adults with PTLD. Treatment includes reduction of immunosuppression (stopping antimetabolites, aiming for low calcineurin inhibitor (CNI) target levels), surgery, radiation, and chemotherapy. R-CHOP (Rituximab-CHOP) has shown good response in PTLD 1 and 2 studies. Rituximab alone may be used in EBV-driven early PTLD. Compared to CNIs, belatacept has a much higher risk of PTLD, especially in EBV + to − transplants.

Dierickx D, Habermann TM. Post-transplantation lymphoproliferative disorders in adults. N Engl J Med. 2018;378:549–62.

Wojciechowski D, Vincenti F. Belatacept in kidney transplantation. Curr Opin Organ Transplant. 2012;17(6):640–7.

210. B. Azithromycin.

Tacrolimus is metabolized by the small intestinal CYP3A4 enzymes (see Fig). Part of the absorbed drug in intestinal enterocytes are effluxed by P-glycoprotein pumps. Inducers of the CYP3A4 system decrease the tacrolimus level, whereas inhibitors of CYP3A4 increase the tacrolimus level:

Figure representing Drug metabolism of Tacrolimus

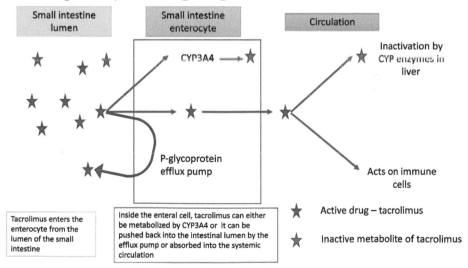

Tacrolimus drug interactions

antibiotics:

    macrolide antibiotics (increase)

    rifampicin (rifampin) (decrease)

    azole antifungal agents (increase)

antiepileptic drugs:

    phenytoin (decrease)

    phenobarbital (decrease)

others:

    danazol (increase)

    cimetidine (increase)

    grapefruit juice (increase)

non-dihydropyridine calcium channel antagonists (increase)

antiretrovirals: protease inhibitors (increase).

Vicari-Christensen M, Repper S, Basile S, *et al.* Tacrolimus: review of pharmacokinetics, pharmacodynamics, and pharmacogenetics to facilitate practitioners' understanding and offer strategies for educating patients and promoting adherence. Prog Transplant. 2009;19(3):277–84.

211. B. Diabetic nephropathy.

The glomeruli in the biopsy show nodular glomerulosclerosis. The nodules are clearly PAS-positive and silver-positive

PAS-positive and silver-positive nodules are seen in diabetic nephropathy and idiopathic nodular glomerulosclerosis. The nodules in diabetes are called Kimmelstiel–Wilson lesions. The differentials for nodular glomerulosclerosis are as follows (see Table 12.2).

Table 12.2 Differential Diagnosis for Nodular Lesions

Lesions	PAS	Silver stain	Congo red
Diabetes mellitus	Positive	Positive	Negative
Idiopathic nodular glomerulosclerosis	Positive	Positive	Negative
Light chain deposition disease	Positive	Negative	Positive
Amyloid	Negative	Negative	Negative
Fibronectin	Positive	Negative	Negative
Collagen	Negative	Negative	Negative

Alsaad KO, Herzenberg AM. Distinguishing diabetic nephropathy from other causes of glomerulosclerosis: an update. J Clin Pathol. 2007;60(1):18–26.

212. C. Calcineurin inhibitor toxicity.

ABO-incompatible transplants undergo the process of accommodation over time. Rising ABO titres in an ABO-incompatible transplant are significant in the initial 2 weeks. HLA DQ and DP have poor endothelial cell expression and are less pathogenic. An MFI level of >2000 would be considered significant. Calcineurin inhibitor toxicity can have varied biopsy findings, including near-normal glomeruli.

1. Functional CNI toxicity:
   a. no changes noticed in the renal biopsy; mediated by afferent arteriolar vasoconstriction
2. Tubular CNI toxicity:
   a. acute:
      i. isometric vacuolization of the proximal tubules
      ii. large cytoplasmic granules (megamitochondria: ciclosporin toxicity; lysosomes in tacrolimus toxicity)
   b. chronic
   i. striped fibrosis
3. Vascular CNI toxicity:
   a. acute:
      i. loss of definition of smooth muscles, cytoplasmic vacuolization
      ii. Thrombotic Microangiopathy (TMA)
   b. chronic:
      i. nodular hyalinization of arteriolar walls
4. Glomerulopathy:
   a. Acute and chronic TMA.

Colvin RB, Chang A (eds). *Diagnostic Pathology: Kidney Diseases*, 3rd edition. Philadelphia, PA: Elsevier, 2019.

213. A. CT angiography.

Transplant renal artery stenosis (TRAS) presents with worsening renal function and hypertension. It is also associated with post-transplant erythrocytosis. It can occur 3 months to 2 years post-transplant. However, most cases are seen in the first 6 months. Doppler ultrasound is commonly used as a screening tool for TRAS, whereas angiography provides a definitive diagnosis. Endovascular therapy with percutaneous transluminal angioplasty and drug-eluting stent placement results in improved BP control and graft function.

Chen W, Kayler LK, Zand MS, et al. Transplant renal artery stenosis: clinical manifestations, diagnosis and therapy. Clin Kidney J. 2015;8(1):71–8.

214. E. Transplant glomerulopathy.

Chronic antibody mediated rejection (AMR) is a condition in which histological evidence of chronic injury is related to DSA interaction with the vascular endothelium. GBM double contouring is a histological feature of chronic AMR. There may be an active component, in addition, if chronic changes are associated with microcirculatory inflammation such as glomerulitis, peritubular capillaritis, or endothelial cell inflammation. Pulsed steroids can be given to treat the active component. The mainstay of treatment for chronic AMR is optimizing maintenance immunosuppression. Recurrent primary FSGS is unlikely to occur 10 years post-renal transplant. It usually occurs early, even days, post-transplant. Interstitial fibrosis and tubular atrophy can explain the proteinuria, but not the histological changes. Taking into consideration the DSA and time post-transplant, transplant glomerulopathy, rather than *de novo* MPGN, is more likely.

Garces JC, Giusti S, Staffeld- Coit C, et al. Antibody- mediated rejection: a review. Ochsner J. 2017;17(1):46–55.

215. C. Passenger lymphocyte syndrome.

TMA in a renal transplant can be *de novo* or recurrent. aHUS is usually a defect in the alternate complement pathway leading to TMA. Membrane cofactor protein mutation has a lower risk of recurrence (20%), compared to *CFH* gene mutation (75%) and CFB mutation (100%). Eculizumab therapy is useful in treating aHUS and also in prevention of TMA in the graft in a patient with aHUS. Drugs such as tacrolimus, ciclosporin, everolimus, sirolimus, and valaciclovir are associated with TMA. The combination of tacrolimus and sirolimus is known to carry a high risk of TMA, and its combined use is discouraged. Accelerated hypertension can also cause TMA and graft dysfunction. AMR is unlikely with negative C4d.

Mundra VRR, Mannon RB. Thrombotic microangiopathy in a transplant recipient. Clin J Am Soc Nephrol. 2018;13(8):1251–3.

Noris M, Remuzzi G. Thrombotic microangiopathy after kidney transplantation. Am J Transplant. 2010;10(7):1517–23.

Take-Home Messages

1. Reduction of immunosuppression is the first line of treatment for BK viraemia.
2. The risk of ESRD in potential live donors is high in Afro-Caribbeans, those with a family history of renal disease, and the young. Genetic testing is recommended for potential live donors with a family history of kidney disease. The absolute risk remains low.
3. Cellular or T cell-mediated rejection is treated with pulsed methylprednisolone. Steroid-resistant cases can be treated with ATG or alemtuzumab. AMR can be treated with IVIg, plasma exchange, or rituximab.
4. SPK transplants would offer better survival, compared to kidney transplants alone, in those fit to undergo the procedure. Patients need to have a good cardiovascular status. Type 2 diabetics can also undergo SPK transplant based on certain criteria.
5. Active cancer or infection is an absolute contraindication for transplantation. Provided patients have been treated and are disease-free for a defined period, they can undergo transplantation. Waiting time following treatment can range from 2 to 5 years, based on the type and stage of cancer.
6. Immunosuppressed patients are at high risk of COVID-19. Those on immunosuppression have a poor antibody response to vaccination.
7. ABO subgroup A2 expresses lower levels of A antigen on the cell surface and is less immunogenic towards anti-A immunoglobulin present in blood group O or B recipients. A2 to O or A2 to B with titres <1:8 would be low immunological risk, with no need for additional immunosuppression. For immunologically incompatible transplants, enrolling pairs in the paired exchange scheme would offer the best possibility of finding a compatible donor.
8. Anti-proliferatives, such as mycophenolate and azathioprine, are stopped when patients return to dialysis following graft failure. CNIs are best to be continued in order to maintain residual renal function. Prednisolone, if to be withdrawn, should be tapered by 1 mg per month. If patients are likely to be transplanted in the following year, then continuing all immunosuppression would reduce allosensitization.
9. Altruistic donors are encouraged to enrol in the paired exchange scheme; however, they can donate to recipients with no genetic or emotional relationship.
10. Graft intolerance syndrome can occur in failing grafts. Once infection is ruled out, a steroid pulse is indicated. Graft nephrectomy can be performed once symptoms are controlled.

11. Renin angiotensin system inhibition is the first-line management of patients with post-transplant erythrocytosis.

12. CMV prophylaxis can be either drug prophylaxis, with valganciclovir as the drug of choice, or pre-emptive therapy which involves regular monitoring with CMV PCR. Mild to moderate CMV disease can be treated with valganciclovir, with severe disease requiring IV ganciclovir.

13. Recurrent disease is the third commonest cause of graft loss, after death with graft function and acute rejection.

14. PTLD can occur many years following transplantation. PTLD occurring in the first 2 years post-transplant is usually EBV-driven. Any patient with weight loss following transplantation should be evaluated for malignancy. Treatment is reduction of immunosuppression and the R-CHOP regimen. In some cases, rituximab alone may be sufficient.

15. Calcineurin inhibitors are metabolized by CYP3A4 enzymes in the gut. Drugs interacting with this enzyme alter the drug levels. Fluconazole, diltiazem, and macrolide antibiotics are common drugs that inhibit the enzymes and cause elevation of tacrolimus levels. Antiretrovirals can also have significant interactions.

16. Recurrent diabetic nephropathy can be related to use of CNIs and mTORi. Tacrolimus is more diabetogenic, compared to ciclosporin.

17. CNIs can cause acute and chronic nephrotoxicity. Biopsy features are non-specific and can include isometric vacuolization, striped fibrosis, arteriolar hyalinosis, interstitial fibrosis, and tubular atrophy.

18. TRAS should be suspected in patients with hypertension and graft dysfunction in the post-transplant setting. Renal hypoperfusion occurring in TRAS results in activation of the renin–angiotensin–aldosterone system; patients present with worsening hypertension, fluid retention, and allograft dysfunction. It usually occurs within 6 months post-transplant. Doppler ultrasound is used for screening, but CT angiography would give a definite diagnosis.

19. AMR diagnosis requires two out of three criteria: microcirculatory inflammation, DSA, C4d. Chronic AMR is characterized by double contouring of the GBM.

20. Eculizumab (anti-C5a) is used as a prophylactic agent in renal transplant for patients with complement-mediated HUS. The recurrence rate of TMA in this setting is as high as 50%. aHUS has a high recurrence rate. Membrane cofactor protein mutation recurs less commonly. TMA post-transplant can be *de novo* or due to recurrent disease. Drugs, viral infections, AMR, and hypertension can all cause *de novo* TMA.

chapter 13

RENAL DISORDERS IN PREGNANCY

QUESTIONS

216. A 28-year-old woman who is 20 weeks into her second pregnancy attended her first routine antenatal appointment with her midwife. She had suffered pain in her lower back for the last 2 weeks. She had no significant past history and her first pregnancy was uneventful.

On examination, her BP was 112/70 mmHg (booking BP 126/76 mmHg). Urinalysis showed protein 3+.

Investigations:

serum creatinine	47 µmol/L (60–110)
serum creatinine (pre-pregnancy)	64 µmol/L (60–110)
urine protein:creatinine ratio	30 mg/mmol (<30)
ultrasound scan of kidneys	normal-sized kidneys, dilatation of the right collecting system

What is the most appropriate next management step?

A. CT KUB
B. IV urography
C. renal biopsy
D. refer to the urology clinic
E. routine antenatal care

Best of Five MCQs for the European Specialty Examination in Nephrology. Shafi Malik, Oxford University Press.
© Oxford University Press 2024. DOI: 10.1093/oso/9780192844163.003.0025

217. **A 29-year-old woman who had undergone a renal transplant 1 year ago attended for a prenatal review. She was trying to conceive and had stopped her contraception. She had a past history of hypertension, chronic rhinitis, and SLE, and was taking ramipril, tacrolimus, simvastatin, mycophenolate mofetil, hydroxychloroquine, and prednisolone.**

On examination, her BP was 104/52 mmHg.

Investigations:

serum urea	6.4 mmol/L (2.5–7.0)
serum creatinine	122 µmol/L (60–110)
urine protein:creatinine ratio	209 mg/mmol (<30)

What would be the most appropriate next step?

A. stop ramipril
B. stop simvastatin
C. stop tacrolimus
D. stop hydroxychloroquine
E. stop mycophenolate mofetil

218. **A 28-year-old woman who had undergone a renal transplant 8 months previously wanted to discuss contraception at her routine clinic review.**

Which of the following would you recommend?

A. barrier methods
B. copper coil
C. combined pill
D. progesterone-only pill
E. oestrogen-containing contraception

219. **A 31-year-old woman who is 12 weeks pregnant attended the antenatal clinic for a scan. She felt very well and had a past history of recurrent urinary tract infections and also a previous miscarriage at 14 weeks 2 years ago. She has had one episode of urinary tract infection during this pregnancy. She asks if she will need antibiotic treatment during the remainder of her pregnancy.**

Urinalysis showed protein 2++, blood 1+, leukocytes 3+, nitrites +ve.

What would be the most appropriate course of action?

A. commence cranberry juice
B. commence IV antibiotics
C. commence prophylactic antibiotics
D. commence sodium hyaluronate
E. ultrasound scan of kidneys

220. **A 29-year-old woman was seen in the renal outpatient clinic. She had undergone a renal transplant 15 years ago and was taking tacrolimus, mycophenolate, and candesartan. She was trying to conceive and wanted to discuss the implications of a pregnancy.**

Investigations:

serum urea	9.8 mmol/L (2.5–7.0)
serum creatinine	198 µmol/L (60–110)
eGFR	27 mL/min/1.73 m²
urine protein:creatinine ratio	54.3 mg/mmol (<30)

What would be the most appropriate pre-conception advice to give her?

A. pregnancy is contraindicated

B. risk of preterm birth, probably with low birthweight

C. start anticoagulation and continue until after delivery

D. start aspirin at the time of conception to prevent pre-eclampsia

E. tacrolimus should be switched to sirolimus

221. **A 36-year-old woman attended the obstetrics–nephrology clinic at 26 weeks in her second pregnancy. She had a past history of IgA nephropathy and hypertension, and was taking labetalol and iron tablets.**

On examination, her BP was 125/83 mmHg.

Investigations:

serum creatinine	44 µmol/L (60–110)
serum urea	3.4 mmol/L (2.5–7.0)
haemoglobin	129 g/L (130–180)
urine protein:creatinine ratio	66.7 mg/mmol (<30)
fetal ultrasound scan	normal fetal growth

What would be the next best step?

A. doxazosin

B. methyldopa

C. nifedipine

D. no change

E. thiazide diuretic

222. **A 23-year-old woman with CKD attended the obstetrics–nephrology clinic for review when she was 16 weeks pregnant. She was feeling well, and her observations were normal.**

Investigations:
serum urea	9.8 mmol/L (2.5–7.0)
serum creatinine	243 µmol/L (60–110)
serum potassium	4.0 mmol/L (3.5–4.9)
serum bicarbonate	22 mmol/L (20–28)

When would you recommend this patient to start dialysis?

A. haemodialysis when the serum creatinine level rises above 250 µmol/L

B. haemodialysis when the serum urea level rises above 17 mmol/L

C. haemodialysis when the serum urea level rises above 25 mmol/L

D. haemodialysis when uraemic symptoms develop

E. peritoneal dialysis when the serum urea level rises above 20 mmol/L

223. **A 38-year-old woman is seen in the renal transplant clinic. She had undergone a renal transplant 18 months previously. She was well and reported being 10 weeks pregnant. She was taking azathioprine, amlodipine, candesartan, metformin, and tacrolimus.**

On examination, she was overweight and her BP was 108/72 mmHg.

Investigations:
serum urea	7.0 mmol/L (2.5–7.0)
serum creatinine	120 µmol/L (60–110)
urine protein:creatinine ratio	150 mg/mmol (<30)
blood tacrolimus (trough)	6.2 nmol/L (8.0–12.0)

What is the most appropriate next step?

A. stop azathioprine

B. stop amlodipine

C. stop candesartan

D. stop metformin

E. stop tacrolimus

224. **A 37-year-old lady attended the antenatal clinic for the first time when she was 14 weeks pregnant. She has a history of recurrent urinary tract infections.**

On examination, her BP was 108/72 mmHg.
Urinalysis showed blood 2+, protein 3+.

Investigations:

serum urea	5.4 mmol/L (2.5–7.0)
serum creatinine	118 µmol/L (60–110)
urine protein:creatinine ratio	154 mg/mmol (<30)
antinuclear antibodies	negative
anti-double-stranded DNA (ELISA) antibodies	15 U/mL (<73)

What is the most appropriate next step?

A. PLA2R antibody
B. platelet-derived growth factor
C. renal biopsy
D. factor Xa level
E. ultrasound scan of kidneys

225. **A 35-year-old woman attended the antenatal clinic and was found to have proteinuria at 17 weeks' gestation in her first pregnancy. She had no significant past history. Her mother had early-onset pre-eclampsia during her pregnancies.**

On examination, her BP was 125/82 mmHg and she had marked swelling of her ankles up her knees.

Investigations:

serum urea	5.3 mmol/L (2.5–7.0)
serum creatinine	66 µmol/L (60–110)
serum albumin	26 g/L (37–49)
urine protein:creatinine ratio	937 mg/mmol (<30)
antinuclear antibodies	1:160 dilution (negative at 1:20)
serum complement C3	57 mg/dL (65–190)
anti-double-stranded DNA (ELISA) antibodies	12 U/mL (<73)
ultrasound scan of kidneys	normal-sized kidneys, with mild dilatation of the pelvicalyceal system on the right

What is the most appropriate next step in investigation?

A. PLA2R antibody
B. platelet-derived growth factor
C. renal biopsy
D. THSD7A
E. anti-cardiolipin antibody

226. A 36-year-old woman attended the antenatal clinic and was found to have proteinuria at 11 weeks' gestation in her second pregnancy. She had a past history of type 2 diabetes and hypertension. She had pre-eclampsia diagnosed in her first pregnancy 4 years ago. She was taking aspirin, folic acid, metformin, and nifedipine.

> **On examination, her BP was 130/80 mmHg.**

> Investigations:

> | | |
> |---|---|
> | serum urea | 7.0 mmol/L (2.5–7.0) |
> | serum creatinine | 140 µmol/L (60–110) |
> | serum cholesterol | 8.9 mmol/L (<5.2) |
> | urine protein:creatinine ratio | 820 mg/mmol (<30) |

What is the most important next step in management?

A. aspirin
B. canagliflozin
C. candesartan
D. dalteparin
E. simvastatin

227. A 32-year-old woman attended the antenatal clinic and was found to have isolated proteinuria at 12 weeks' gestation in her first pregnancy. Her mother had early-onset pre-eclampsia during her pregnancies.

> **On examination, her BP was 144/89 mmHg.**

> Investigations:

> | | |
> |---|---|
> | serum urea | 5.3 mmol/L (2.5–7.0) |
> | serum creatinine | 66 µmol/L (60–110) |
> | serum albumin | 29 g/L (37–49) |
> | urine protein:creatinine ratio | 150 mg/mmol (<30) |

What is the most appropriate next step in management?

A. aspirin
B. doxazosin
C. folic acid
D. dalteparin
E. labetalol

228. **A 37-year-old lady with CKD due to APKD had a renal transplant 6 months previously. She had an episode of acute rejection treated with methylprednisolone in the third month post-transplant, and was taking tacrolimus, azathioprine, felodipine, and prednisolone. She was well and wished to consider a pregnancy as soon as possible.**

On examination, her BP was 108/72 mmHg.

Investigations:

serum creatinine	127 μmol/L (60–110)
urine protein:creatinine ratio	54 mg/mmol (<30)
blood tacrolimus level (trough)	5.4 nmol/L (8.0–12.0)

What is the most important advice to give her?

A. attempt to conceive now

B. delay pregnancy

C. increased risk of rejection during pregnancy

D. switch tacrolimus to ciclosporin

E. will require a caesarean section

229. **A 35-year-old lady with a history of hypertension and diabetes presented to the antenatal clinic for the first time when she was 36 weeks pregnant. She reported feeling unwell.**

On examination, her BP was 200/100 mmHg. She was delivered by emergency caesarean section the following day. Her BP remained high following delivery at 170/100 mmHg.
Urinalysis: negative.

Investigations:

serum urea	10 mmol/L (2.5–7.0)
serum creatinine	300 μmol/L (60–110)
haemoglobin	93 g/L (130–180)
platelet count	90 × 10^9/L (150–400)
serum alanine aminotransferase	29 U/L (5–35)
Ultrasound scan of kidneys	normal-sized kidneys, mild pelvic dilatation in the right kidney

What is the most likely diagnosis?

A. acute glomerulonephritis

B. acute tubular necrosis

C. hydronephrosis

D. HELLP syndrome

E. pre-eclampsia

230. **A 34-year-old woman attended the antenatal clinic for the first time when she was 26 weeks pregnant. She had a past history of early-onset pre-eclampsia in her first pregnancy 5 years previously and was monitoring her BP at home. She was taking aspirin, ferrous sulfate, and folic acid.**

   On examination, her home BP readings were consistently between 136/86 and
   141/96 mmHg.
   Urinalysis showed blood 2+, protein 2+.

   Investigations:

serum urea	7.0 mmol/L (2.5–7.0)
serum creatinine	115 μmol/L (60–110)
urine protein:creatinine ratio	175 mg/mmol (<30)

   ## What is the most appropriate next management step?

   A. amlodipine
   B. bisoprolol
   C. furosemide
   D. lisinopril
   E. methyldopa

216. E. Routine antenatal care.

During pregnancy, the kidney increases in size, by approximately 1 cm, as the volume of blood filtered increases by approximately 70%, owing to the action of hormones, including nitric oxide, prostaglandins, and relaxin. This results in an increase in GFR of approximately 25% and a fall in the serum creatinine concentration. In pregnancy, the estimated GFR underestimates renal function and should not be used.

In addition, in over half of pregnancies, there is marked dilatation of the collecting system as a result of both hormonal and mechanical factors. Under the influence of oestrogen, progesterone, relaxin, and prostaglandin, the collecting system dilates from as early as 8 weeks. Dilatation is much more prominent on the right side due to anatomical dextrorotation of the uterus. The left collecting system is protected from compression by the gas-filled sigmoid colon. Approximately 80% of women will have hydronephrosis by the third trimester.

Renal biopsy here is not indicated as there is no suggestion of glomerular disease. Urine protein excretion increases during the course of normal pregnancy and proteinuria of <300 mg/24 hours is not significant in isolation. Stones are fairly uncommon in pregnancy and usually occur in women with pre-existing stone disease, and this patient has no microscopic haematuria. The back pain can be attributed to symphysis pubis dysfunction, given the insidious onset and also the current gestation. IV urography and CT KUB would be giving unnecessary radiation exposure.

Section VII. Pregnancy and renal disease. In: RJ Johnson, J Feehally, J Floege, eds. *Comprehensive Clinical Nephrology*, 6th edition. St Louis, MO: Elsevier, 2015. https://www.us.elsevierhealth.com/comprehens ive-clinical-nephrology-9780323479097.html

Jeyabalan A, Lain KY. Anatomic and functional changes of the upper urinary tract during pregnancy. Urol Clin North Am. 2007;34:1–6.

217. E. Stop mycophenolate mofetil.

Pregnancy after renal transplantation must be carefully planned. It is recommended that women wait for 1 year post-transplant to attempt conception, provided that they have stable graft function and no recent rejection episodes. Mycophenolate mofetil has been shown to be teratogenic, causing congenital malformations such as ear defects, short digits, hypoplastic nails, deafness, and cleft palate. It is also associated with an increased risk of spontaneous miscarriage. Therefore, mycophenolate mofetil should be switched to an alternative, such as azathioprine, 3 months before conception in order to monitor graft function. Other immunosuppressants that are teratogenic and need to be stopped pre-conception are methotrexate and cyclophosphamide. Those that are generally considered safe in pregnancy are prednisolone, azathioprine, ciclosporin, tacrolimus, and hydroxychloroquine.

Sifontis NM, Coscia LA, Constantinescu S, et al. Pregnancy outcomes in solid organ transplant recipients with exposure to mycophenolate mofetil or sirolimus. Transplantation. 2006;82:1698–702.

Wiles K, Chappell L, Clark K, et al. Clinical practice guideline on pregnancy and renal disease. BMC Nephrol. 2019;20(1):401.

218. D. Progesterone-only pill.

CKD reduces fertility, but women with CKD can still have an unintended pregnancy. Safe and effective contraception is important, as there are significant risks associated with unplanned pregnancy (including risks from potentially teratogenic medications).

There is a risk of hypertension, thromboembolism, and cervical cancer with oestrogen-containing contraception, especially in women with pre-existing relevant comorbidities such as hypertension. In transplant recipients, oestrogen has also been shown to interfere with calcineurin inhibitor metabolism which can affect graft function adversely.

These risks are not seen with the progesterone-only pill (mini pill), progesterone-containing intrauterine system (Mirena®), and progesterone subdermal implant (Nexplanon®); hence they are considered the safest. Some studies stipulate a risk of breast malignancy, but data are insufficient.

Non-hormonal methods, such as the copper coil, can be used, but there is concern around lower efficacy and infection in immunosuppressed patients. Barrier contraception is fairly effective and good at prevention of sexually transmitted infections, but 18–21% of couples conceive within the first year of using condoms; hence they are not considered reliable enough. There is varied information about failure rates for various contraceptive methods, but overall, failure rates for the contraceptive pill, implant, and progesterone-containing intrauterine device (Mirena®) are 9%, 0.2%, and 0.05%, respectively, within the first year of use, suggesting progesterone-only methods to be the most effective.

Estes CM, Westhoff C. Contraception for the transplant patient. Semin Perinatol. 2007;31:372–7.

Wiles K, Chappell L, Clark K, et al. Clinical practice guideline on pregnancy and renal disease. BMC Nephrol. 2019;20(1):401.

219. C. Commence prophylactic antibiotics.

Physiological collecting system dilatation occurs in pregnancy, leading to urinary stasis, slow emptying, and potentially reflux, all of which predispose pregnant women to bacteriuria and subsequently a higher risk of asymptomatic infection that may progress to development of symptomatic ascending infection (acute pyelonephritis). Glycosuria will also help with bacterial growth. Bacteriuria warrants prompt assessment and treatment, even when asymptomatic, because of an increased risk of ascending infection, bacteraemia, septic shock, renal failure, or spontaneous miscarriage.

Guidelines recommend that women with reflux nephropathy, congenital anomalies of the kidneys and urinary tract, CKD and/or taking immunosuppression, and a history of recurrent UTIs should be offered antibiotic prophylaxis during pregnancy after a single UTI in pregnancy, including asymptomatic bacteriuria. Cranberry juice is not indicated and there is no role for ultrasound in this instance. Sodium hyaluronate is used for treatment of recurrent cystitis. The patient does not have features of pyelonephritis, so there is no indication for IV antibiotics. It is also recommended that if a woman was taking prophylaxis pre-conception, it should be continued in pregnancy using agents that are considered safe. Antibiotics considered safe to use for treatment of UTIs are penicillins, cephalosporins, and fosfomycin. Trimethoprim is not safe in the first trimester but can be used from the second trimester onwards. Nitrofurantoin can be used earlier in pregnancy, but not in the third trimester, as evidence suggests an increased risk of neonatal jaundice. Nitrofurantoin is also ineffective if pre-pregnancy eGFR was <45 mL/min.

National Institute for Health and Care Excellence (2018). Urinary tract infection (recurrent): antimicrobial prescribing. NICE guideline [NG112]. Available from: https://www.nice.org.uk/guidance/ng112

Parasuraman R, Julian K; AST IDCOP. Urinary tract infections in solid organ transplantation. Am J Transplant. 2013;1(Suppl 4):327–36.

Smaill FM, Vazquez JC. Antibiotics for asymptomatic bacteriuria in pregnancy. Cochrane Database Syst Rev. 2015;8:CD000490. doi:10.1002/14651858.CD000490.pub3. Update in: Cochrane Database Syst Rev. 2019 Nov 25;2019(11): PMID: 26252501.

Wiles K, Chappell L, Clark K, et al. Clinical practice guideline on pregnancy and renal disease. BMC Nephrol. 2019;20(1):401.

In: J Barratt, P Topham, S Carr, M Arici, A Liew, eds. *Oxford Desk Reference Nephrology*, 2nd edition. 2021; pp. 402–32.

220. B. Risk of preterm baby, probably with low birthweight.

Current recommendations advise CKD patients are given information prior to conception about possible risks of pregnancy to the mother and baby. Potential complications in pregnancy include pre-eclampsia, impact on graft function, and possible early delivery resulting in a baby with a low birthweight. The risks of an adverse pregnancy outcome in this patient with moderately impaired renal transplant function and hypertension would be significant, with an increased risk of pre-eclampsia and preterm birth. Although mycophenolate and candesartan are contraindicated in pregnancy, tacrolimus can be safely continued. Sirolimus is not recommended in pregnancy. Use of aspirin to reduce the risk of pre-eclampsia is recommended to start at 12 weeks of pregnancy. Anticoagulation is recommended for patients with nephrotic proteinuria (or other thromboembolic risk factors) and is generally continued for 6 weeks into the post partum period.

Wiles K, Chappell L, Clark K, et al. Clinical practice guideline on pregnancy and renal disease. BMC Nephrol. 2019;20(1):401.

221. D. No change.

This patient's BP is under control and within the acceptable range. Based on the CHIPS trial, patients with tight BP control (diastolic target <85 mmHg) had fewer frequent episodes of severe hypertension (>160/110 mmHg). A post-hoc analysis of the same trial showed severe hypertension was associated with a higher probability of pregnancy loss, low birthweight, pre-eclampsia, preterm delivery, and abnormal platelets and liver enzymes.

Magee LA, von Dadelszen P, Rey E, et al. Less-tight versus tight control of hypertension in pregnancy. N Engl J Med. 2015;372(5):407–17.

Magee LA, von Dadelszen P, Singer J, et al. The CHIPS randomized controlled trial (Control of Hypertension in Pregnancy Study): is severe hypertension just an elevated blood pressure? Hypertension. 2016;68(5):1153–9.

222. B. Haemodialysis when the serum urea level rises above 17 mmol/L.

The UK Renal Association recommends initiation and maintenance of dialysis in patients with kidney disease, based on urea concentrations and residual kidney function, along with gestation, renal function trajectory, fluid balance, biochemical parameters, BP, and uraemic symptoms. The guidelines suggest starting dialysis when the urea concentration is >17 mmol/L and maintaining a pre-dialysis urea concentration of <12.5 mmol/L. Haemodialysis should be modified, so women might receive long and frequent sessions. An alternative approach to increase the weekly hours of dialysis is to base the therapy on biochemical parameters (pre-dialysis urea concentration). Although the guidelines mention the general term 'biochemical parameters', it would include creatinine, potassium, and bicarbonate concentrations. Evidence shows that the best parameter to monitor and adjust dialysis adequacy is urea concentration, as mid-week pre-dialysis concentrations of <12.5 mmol/L are discriminatory in determining successful pregnancy outcome. Use of other clearance calculations (including Kt/V) is not recommended.

Wiles K, Chappell L, Clark K, *et al*. Clinical practice guideline on pregnancy and renal disease. BMC Nephrol. 2019;20(1):401.

223. C. Stop candesartan.

ACE inhibitors can be continued until conception and should be discontinued from the second trimester onwards as they are fetotoxic. ARBs should be discontinued pre-conception as there are insufficient safety data on their effects in early pregnancy. Candesartan should be stopped in this case, and the BP monitored. Metformin, amlodipine, and azathioprine can be continued in pregnancy.

Bateman BT, Patorno E, Desai RJ, *et al*. Angiotensin-converting enzyme inhibitors and the risk of congenital malformations. Obstet Gynecol. 2017;129:174–84.

In: J Barratt, P Topham, S Carr, M Arici, A Liew, eds. *Oxford Desk Reference Nephrology*, 2nd edition. 2021; pp. 402–32.

224. E. Ultrasound scan of kidneys.

This patient should have a renal ultrasound scan to assess the size and structure. Given the history of recurrent urinary tract infections, mild renal impairment, and proteinuria, chronic pyelonephritis and reflux are likely. It would be important to establish if the renal function is deteriorating rapidly and if she would fit the criteria for a biopsy during pregnancy.

Brunskill N. Renal biopsy in pregnancy. In: K Bramham, M Hall, C Nelson-Piercy, eds. *Renal Disease in Pregnancy*, 2nd edition. Cambridge: Cambridge University Press, 2018; pp. 216–20.

In: J Barratt, P Topham, S Carr, M Arici, A Liew, eds. *Oxford Desk Reference Nephrology*, 2nd edition. 2021; pp. 402–32.

Wiles K, Chappell L, Clark K, *et al*. Clinical practice guideline on pregnancy and renal disease. BMC Nephrol. 2019;20(1):401.

225. C. Renal biopsy.

A renal biopsy can be technically difficult to perform in pregnancy if the patient is unable to lie in the usual prone position. Small studies have shown the risk of bleeding post-biopsy is higher in pregnancy, especially between 23 and 28 weeks (7% antenatally vs 1% postnatally). Therefore, it is important to perform a renal biopsy during the first or early second trimester (before 22 weeks) and where the histological diagnosis could change the patient's management during pregnancy. In this patient, severe symptomatic nephrotic syndrome at 17 weeks would be an indication for a biopsy, as it could lead to management change.

Brunskill N. Renal biopsy in pregnancy. In: K Bramham, M Hall, C Nelson-Piercy, eds. *Renal Disease in Pregnancy*, 2nd edition. Cambridge: Cambridge University Press, 2018; pp. 216–20.

Wiles K, Chappell L, Clark K, *et al*. Clinical practice guideline on pregnancy and renal disease. BMC Nephrol. 2019;20(1):401.

226. D. Dalteparin.

The presence of significant proteinuria (PCR >300 mg/mmol) or nephrotic syndrome is associated with an increased risk of thromboembolism in pregnancy. In the absence of any contraindication, women are offered thromboprophylaxis for safety with low-molecular weight heparin during pregnancy and for 6 weeks post-partum. In women with lower levels of proteinuria, it is important to consider this as an additional thromboembolic risk factor when considering whether a woman should receive thromboprophylaxis during pregnancy. Simvastatin, SGLT2 inhibitors, and ARBs are contraindicated in pregnancy. Aspirin to reduce the risk of pre-eclampsia is recommended to be started at 12 weeks' gestation.

Royal College of Obstetricians and Gynaecologists (2015). Reducing the risk of venous thromboembolism during pregnancy and the puerperium. Green-top guideline No. 37a. Available from: https://www.rcog.org.uk/globalassets/documents/guidelines/gtg-37a.pdf

In: J Barratt, P Topham, S Carr, M Arici, A Liew, eds. *Oxford Desk Reference Nephrology*, 2nd edition. 2021; pp. 310–15.

Wiles K, Chappell L, Clark K, et al. Clinical practice guideline on pregnancy and renal disease. BMC Nephrol. 2019;20(1):401.

227. A. Aspirin.

Pre-eclampsia (PET) affects 3–5% of all pregnancies, and in some studies, 40% of women with CKD are reported to be affected by PET, which is associated with increased maternal and fetal morbidity and mortality. In high-risk populations, aspirin (75–150 mg daily) has been shown to reduce the risk of pre-eclampsia and it is now recommended that aspirin prophylaxis is considered in women with renal disease.

In: J Barratt, P Topham, S Carr, M Arici, A Liew, eds. *Oxford Desk Reference Nephrology*, 2nd edition. 2021; pp. 402–32.

Rolnik DL, Wright D, Poon LC, et al. Aspirin versus placebo in pregnancies at high risk for preterm preeclampsia. N Engl J Med. 2017;377(7):613–22.

Hypertension in pregnancy: diagnosis and management. NICE guideline [NG133]. Published: 25 June 2019. Available from: https://www.nice.org.uk/guidance/ng133

Wiles K, Chappell L, Clark K, et al. Clinical practice guideline on pregnancy and renal disease. BMC Nephrol. 2019;20(1):401.

228. B. Delay pregnancy.

Women are usually advised to defer pregnancy for approximately 12 months post-transplant. The optimal time for pregnancy post-transplant is between 1 and 5 years and when a woman is at lower risk of transplant complications and is stable on medicines that are safe in pregnancy. Women with a renal transplant are at high risk of pre-eclampsia. Registries have reported an incidence of pre-eclampsia of 15–58% in women with a transplant. A woman with a renal transplant will not inevitably need delivery by caesarean section, unless there are specific obstetric indications for a caesarean section. Tacrolimus is safe in pregnancy and there is no benefit in switching to ciclosporin.

Sarween N, Drage M, Car S. Pregnancy and the renal transplant recipient. In: K Bramham, M Hall, C Nelson-Piercy, eds. *Renal Disease in Pregnancy*, 2nd edition. Cambridge: Cambridge University Press, 2018; pp. 120–37.

Wiles K, Chappell L, Clark K, et al. Clinical practice guideline on pregnancy and renal disease. BMC Nephrol. 2019;20(1):401.

229. E. Pre-eclampsia.

Pre-eclampsia occurs in approximately 3–5% of normal pregnancies and is more prevalent in women with CKD. Pre-eclampsia occurs after 20 weeks of pregnancy and is diagnosed when hypertension develops in a previously normotensive woman (measured on two different occasions at least 4 hours apart) and usually in the presence of proteinuria with urine PCR >300 mg/day. Women with CKD often have pre-existing hypertension, proteinuria, and elevated creatinine levels, and it can be very difficult to distinguish from superimposed pre-eclampsia. Pre-eclampsia is associated with endothelial dysfunction and patients may have signs of multisystem involvement, including thrombocytopenia, haemolysis, AKI, liver dysfunction, and cerebral and visual disturbance or uteroplacental dysfunction. A diagnosis of pre-eclampsia can be made in a hypertensive pregnant woman in the absence of proteinuria when there are other systemic features. Recently, abnormalities identified in circulating angiogenic factors (reduction in placental growth factor and an increase in anti-angiogenic factors (soluble fms-like tyrosine kinase-1 (sFlT-1)) have been detected before the onset of pre-eclampsia and explored as potential predictors of pre-eclampsia in normal pregnant women. However, to date, there are little data on pregnant women with CKD.

In: J Barratt, P Topham, S Carr, M Arici, A Liew, eds. *Oxford Desk Reference Nephrology*, 2nd edition. 2021; pp. 402–32.

Wiles K, Chappell L, Clark K, et al. Clinical practice guideline on pregnancy and renal disease. BMC Nephrol. 2019;20(1):401.

230. E. Methyldopa.

It is recommended that BP is maintained at 135/85 mmHg or less in pregnancy. Recommended antihypertensive agents in pregnancy are labetalol, nifedipine, and methyldopa.

ACE-Is and ARBs are contraindicated in pregnancy due to the risk of fetal abnormalities, and should be stopped as soon as pregnancy is diagnosed. Diuretics should be avoided in pregnancy due to the risk of hypoperfusion and fetal harm.

National Institute for Health and Care Excellence (2019). Hypertension in pregnancy: diagnosis and management. NICE guideline [NG133]. Available from: https://www.nice.org.uk/guidance/ng133

In: J Barratt, P Topham, S Carr, M Arici, A Liew, eds. *Oxford Desk Reference Nephrology*, 2nd edition. 2021; pp. 402–32.

Wiles K, Chappell L, Clark K, et al. Clinical practice guideline on pregnancy and renal disease. BMC Nephrol. 2019;20(1):401.

Take-Home Messages

1. Safe and effective contraception is important in women with CKD, as there are significant risks associated with unplanned pregnancy; in transplant recipients, the progesterone-only pill, Mirena® coil, or implants are recommended.
2. Pre-pregnancy counselling is important for women with pre-existing renal disease, to discuss optimal timing of pregnancy and explain any increased maternal or fetal risks; transplant patients should ideally wait for a year post-transplant with stable graft function before they conceive.
3. Before pregnancy (or when a pregnancy is diagnosed), all medications should be reviewed to ensure they are safe to take during pregnancy; tacrolimus and azathioprine are safe in pregnancy, whereas mycophenolate, sirolimus, ACE-Is, and ARBs must be switched to alternatives.

4. Women with renal disease are at high risk of pre-eclampsia and should be offered aspirin prophylaxis at 12 weeks' gestation to reduce the risk of pre-eclampsia. A diagnosis of pre-eclampsia can be made in a hypertensive pregnant woman in the absence of proteinuria when there are other systemic features.

5. BP during pregnancy should be monitored and controlled, according to guidelines and using medications that are safe in pregnancy. Recommended antihypertensive agents in pregnancy are labetalol, nifedipine, and methyldopa.

6. Renal biopsy should only be considered during the first or early second trimester of pregnancy and if the outcome could lead to a change in treatment during the pregnancy.

7. It is recommended to start dialysis in pregnant women when the urea concentration is >17 mmol/L and to maintain a pre-dialysis urea concentration of <12.5 mmol/L.

231. A 53-year-old man, who has been on haemodialysis for 10 years, complains of reduced appetite. Staff are concerned as he looks frailer, and comment that 'his clothes are hanging off him'. He has lost 15% of weight in 6 months, from 100 kg (BMI 24 kg/m^2) to 85 kg (BMI 21 kg/m^2). A recent dietician review noted that his daily average energy and protein intakes are 20 kcal/kg and 0.8 g/kg, respectively.

On examination, he was emaciated, with protruded clavicles and a prominent scapula.

Investigations:
serum phosphate   1.04 mmol/L (0.80–1.45)
serum albumin   31 g/L (37–49)
serum bicarbonate   19 mmol/L (21–29)
serum CRP   18 mg/L (<10)
Kt/V   0.96

Which of the factors can explain this presentation?

A. decreased appetite and dietary intake
B. metabolic acidosis
C. poor dialysis adequacy
D. systemic inflammation
E. all of the above

Best of Five MCQs for the European Specialty Examination in Nephrology. Shafi Malik, Oxford University Press.
© Oxford University Press 2024. DOI: 10.1093/oso/9780192844163.003.0027

232. **A 42-year-old woman on peritoneal dialysis presents to clinic with tiredness and lethargy, and has been unable to walk >50 ft without resting. She gives a 3-month history of bloating, postprandial fullness, and early satiety, and consequently has lost 8% of her body weight.**

> **On examination, she is found to have significant muscle wasting in both upper and lower limbs.**

> Investigations:
> | | |
> |---|---|
> | serum phosphate | 1.49 mmol/L (0.80–1.45) |
> | serum potassium | 3.2 mmol/L (3.5–4.9) |
> | serum total cholesterol | 2.3 mmol/L (<5.2) |
> | serum urea | 2.0 mmol/L (2.5–7.0) |

How would malnutrition be best measured?

A. anthropometry/body composition
B. dietary intake assessment
C. handgrip strength
D. serum albumin
E. Subjective Global Assessment

233. **A 70-year-old woman with CKD stage 3 was admitted to the intensive care unit with septic shock and AKI on CKD. On day 4 of hospitalization, she became oliguric and fluid-overloaded, and was started on continuous renal replacement therapy. There was moderate muscle wasting noticeable on her temporal areas, clavicles, and shoulders.**

What would be the recommended protein intake?

A. 1.8–2.5 g/kg/day
B. 1.3–1.5 g/kg/day
C. 1.5–1.7 g/kg/day
D. 0.8–1.0 g/kg/day
E. 1.0–1.3 g/kg/day

234. **A 60-year-old man with CKD stage 4 is seen in clinic. He has a history of hypertension and hypercholesterolaemia. His current weight is 71 kg (BMI 22.4 kg/m²). His appetite is generally good. However, a recent dietary assessment revealed energy and protein intakes of 25 kcal/kg/day and 0.8 g/kg/day, respectively.**

On examination, there are some signs of muscle wasting and mild oedema of the feet and ankles.

Investigations:
serum phosphate	1.31 mmol/L (0.80–1.45)
serum potassium	4.6 mmol/L (3.5–4.9)
serum albumin	36 g/L (37–49)
total cholesterol	6.4 mmol/L (<5.2)

What protein and energy intake would you recommend to prevent malnutrition and CKD progression?

A. 0.6–0.8 g/kg/day + 30–35 kcal/kg/day

B. 0.55–0.6 g/kg/day + 30–35 kcal/kg/day

C. 0.28–0.43 g/kg/day + ketoanalogue supplements + 30–35 kcal/kg/day

D. A and B are correct

E. B and C are correct

235. **A 29-year-old man underwent a deceased donor renal transplant 6 months ago. He gained 7 kg in that time, going from 65.3 kg (BMI 23.3 kg/m²) to 72.3 kg (BMI of 25.8 kg/m²). Analysis of a 7-day food diary revealed an average energy and protein intake of 40 kcal/kg and 1.4 g/kg, respectively. He has a low dietary fibre intake (14 g/day) and high fat intake, particularly saturated fats (15% of total energy).**

Investigations (taken after 12-hour fast):
random plasma glucose	5.1 mmol/L (3.3–4.4)
fasting serum triglycerides	2.6 mmol/L (0.45–2.30)
serum cholesterol	6.8 mmol/L (<5.2)
serum HDL-cholesterol	0.9 mmol/L (>1.55)
serum LDL-cholesterol	4.7 mmol/L (<3.36)

What would be the next best step in management?

A. diet and low-dose statin

B. diet and maximum-dose statin

C. diet with <7% saturated fats and 20–30 g fibre

D. low-dose statin

E. maximum-dose statin

236. **A 51-year-old woman was admitted to the emergency department after consuming an unknown quantity of screenwash and ibuprofen tablets 8 hours previously. She has a past history of depression, deliberate self-harm, and hypertension, for which she takes mirtazapine and amlodipine.**

On examination, she is alert and conversant; her temperature is 37.9°C, pulse 111 beats/min, BP 113/56 mmHg, and saturation 98% on air.

Investigations:

serum creatinine	689 μmol/L (60–110)
serum ethylene glycol	760 mg/L
pH	7.1 (7.35–7.45)
lactate	10 mmol/L (0.5–1.6)

What is the most appropriate treatment?

A. fomepizole
B. haemodialysis
C. haemofiltration
D. intravenous ethanol
E. intravenous fluids

237. **A 34-year-old gentleman is seen in clinic with joint pain, sweats, and AKI on a background of normal renal function. He has a past history of HIV, hypertension, and asthma. Medications include amlodipine, salbutamol inhaler, abacavir, lamivudine, and dolutegravir.**

On examination, his temperature is 37.7°C, pulse 92 beats/min, and BP 166/91 mmHg.

Investigations:

serum creatinine (baseline)	84 μmol/L (60–110)
serum creatinine	348 μmol/L (60–110)
serum albumin	34 g/L (37–49)
eosinophil count	1.3×10^9/ L (0.04–0.40)
urine albumin:creatinine ratio	91 mg/mmol (<2.5)

What is the likely diagnosis?

A. acute tubular necrosis
B. focal segmental glomerulosclerosis
C. hypertensive nephrosclerosis
D. renal tubular acidosis
E. tubulointerstitial nephritis

238. An 82-year-old gentleman with known stable **CKD** stage 4 is admitted to the acute medical take with a widespread erythematous, blistering skin rash. He is known to have hypertension and gout, for which he takes ramipril and allopurinol. Two days prior, he was started on a new medication for his hypertension. Unfortunately he cannot recall the name of this medication.

> On examination, his temperature was 38.3°C, pulse 132 beats/min, and BP 98/49 mmHg.

> Investigations:
> serum urea   17.6 mmol/L (2.5–7.0)
> serum creatinine   333 µmol/L (60–110)
> serum creatinine (baseline) 204 µmol/L (60–110)
> eosinophil count 1.3×10^9/L (0.04–0.40)

Which medication that was started is likely to explain his presentation?

A. amlodipine
B. bendroflumethiazide
C. furosemide
D. metoprolol
E. spironolactone

239. A 57-year-old woman presented with a swollen, painful right knee. She has a past history of **CKD** stage 3, anorexia nervosa, and osteoarthritis. A knee aspiration revealed turbid fluid, and culture grew *Staphylococcus aureus*. She was started on intravenous flucloxacillin 2 g four times daily. For the pain, she was prescribed intravenous paracetamol 1 g four times daily. The next day, she complained of breathlessness.

> Investigations:
> serum urea   21.6 mmol/L (2.5–7.0)
> serum creatinine   510 µmol/L (60–110)
> pH   7.0 (7.35–7.45)
> lactate   1.2 mmol/L (0.5–1.6)

What is the likely explanation for the findings?

A. high anion gap acidosis
B. normal anion gap acidosis
C. respiratory acidosis
D. type A lactic acidosis
E. type B lactic acidosis

240. An 81-year-old woman with CKD stage 4 due to diabetic nephropathy is seen in the renal clinic. She has a past history of moderate left ventricular systolic dysfunction and poorly controlled diabetes. Medications are gliclazide 160 mg twice daily ramipril 10 mg once daily, bisoprolol 10 mg once daily and simvastatin 20 mg once daily

Investigations:
serum creatinine	181 µmol/L (60–110)
eGFR	28 mL/min/1.73 m² (>60)
urine albumin:creatinine ratio	185 mg/mmol (<2.5)
haemoglobin A1c	92 mmol/mol (20–42)

What is the next best management step?

A. dapagliflozin
B. glargine
C. metformin
D. saxagliptin
E. semaglutide

241. An 88-year-old man with CKD stage 5 secondary to diabetic nephropathy has opted for conservative management. He has severe and debilitating back pain radiating to both legs and is bed-bound. MRI of the whole spine demonstrates severe degenerative changes from L3 to L5. He contacted the CKD nurses due to increasing back pain, as paracetamol 1 g four times daily and gabapentin 300 mg once daily were not controlling the pain.

Investigations:
eGFR	13 mL/min/1.73 m² (>60)
serum potassium	6.1 mmol/L (3.5–4.9)
serum adjusted calcium	2.22 mmol/L (2.20–2.60)

What is the next best management step?

A. increase the dose of gabapentin
B. NSAIDs
C. oxycodone
D. refer for surgical opinion
E. refer to the pain team

242. **An 89-year-old patient on haemodialysis suffers a significant hypotensive episode (75/46 mmHg) causing loss of consciousness. There have been similar episodes recently. Over the past 6 months, he has been declining with reduced physical function, increasing frailty, and weight loss. He has a past history of heart failure with reduced ejection fraction of 15% and has been on haemodialysis for 10 years.**

On examination of his chest, there were fine bibasal crepitations.

What is the best management step?

A. add fludrocortisone

B. critical care team for inotropic support

C. discuss end-of-life care with the patient and family

D. fluid resuscitation and review

E. switch to peritoneal dialysis

243. **An 87-year-old woman with CKD stage 5 has opted for conservative management. She has diabetic nephropathy on insulin, and requires four antihypertensive agents to manage her BP and ischaemic heart disease. She complains of severe whole-body itching, with no accompanying rash. Emollients have not provided any relief.**

Investigations:

serum urea	21 mmol/L (2.5–7.0)
serum phosphate	1.3 mmol/L (0.80–1.45)
serum adjusted calcium	2.34 mmol/L (2.20–2.60)

What is the next best step?

A. antihistamines

B. evening primrose oil

C. gabapentin

D. phosphate binders

E. refer to dermatologist

244. **A 67-year-old gentleman on haemodialysis is admitted with pneumonia. He has a past history of severe peripheral vascular disease and COPD on home oxygen. His individualized advanced care plan states he is not for resuscitation and is for ward-based care. Despite best ward-based care, he deteriorates. Following a discussion with him and his family, he is commenced on a palliative care pathway.**

What is the most appropriate next step?

A. subcutaneous midazolam and alfentanil PRN

B. subcutaneous midazolam and hyoscine butylbromide PRN

C. subcutaneous midazolam PRN

D. subcutaneous midazolam, alfentanil, and hyoscine butylbromide PRN

E. syringe driver with midazolam and hyoscine butylbromide

245. **A 73-year-old man with a failing third renal transplant attends the low clearance clinic. His eGFR has been stable for 3 months and he has opted for conservative management. His serum potassium levels are persistently above 6.5 mmol/L. He has been reviewed by a renal dietician and is adhering to low potassium dietary restrictions. His current medications include low-dose prednisolone, tacrolimus and amlodipine.**

Investigations:

serum potassium	6.4 mmol/L (3.5–4.9)
eGFR	10 mL/min/1.73 m^2 (>60)
serum bicarbonate	23 mmol/L (21–29)

What is the next best step to address hyperkalaemia?

A. dialysis

B. dietician review

C. fludrocortisone

D. patiromer

E. sodium bicarbonate

231. E. All of the above.

Malnutrition (specifically protein–energy wasting) in dialysis patients cannot be explained by insufficient nutrient/dietary intake alone. It is instead the result of an interaction between multiple ESRD-related mechanisms, including uraemic toxicity due to poor dialysis adequacy, poor appetite (leading to inadequate dietary intake), dialysis-induced nutrient losses, metabolic acidosis, systemic inflammation, oxidative stress, and physical inactivity.

Carrero JJ, Stenvinkel P, Cuppari L, et al. Etiology of the protein-energy wasting syndrome in chronic kidney disease: a consensus statement from the International Society of Renal Nutrition and Metabolism (ISRNM). J Ren Nutr. 2013;23(2):77–90.

232. E. Subjective Global Assessment.

Several methods are used to assess nutritional status in the dialysis population (e.g. body composition, biochemistry, dietary intake, functional parameters), but the use of a single marker to diagnose malnutrition is subject to the influence of non-nutritional factors, and therefore inappropriate. The 2020 KDOQI nutrition guidelines have recommended the use of the Subjective Global Assessment, a comprehensive nutritional assessment tool which combines different nutritional parameters to minimize the limitations of these methods when used in isolation.

Ikizler TA, Cuppari L. The 2020 updated KDOQI Clinical Practice Guidelines for nutrition in chronic kidney disease. Blood Purif. 2021;50(4–5):667–71.

233. C. 1.5–1.7 g/kg/day.

The recommended protein intake in AKI depends on the individual's catabolic state and type of RRT as follows:

Non-catabolic/no RRT	Catabolic/no RRT	Catabolic/IHD	Catabolic/CRRT
0.8–1.0 g/kg/day	1.0–1.3 g/kg/day	1.3–1.5 g/kg/day	1.5–1.7 g/kg/day

RRT, Renal Replacement Therapy; IHD, intermittent haemodialysis; CRRT, Continous Renal Replacement Therapy.

Fiaccadori E, Sabatino A, Barazzoni R, et al. ESPEN guideline on clinical nutrition in hospitalized patients with acute or chronic kidney disease. Clin Nutr. 2021;40(4):1644–68.

234. E. B and C are correct.

The updated 2020 KDOQI nutrition guidelines recommend that protein restriction (0.55–0.6 or 0.28–0.43 g/kg/day with ketoanalogues) should be implemented in people with non diabetic CKD stages 3 & 4 who are metabolically stable to slow CKD progression. Implementation of these low/very low-protein diets should be done under close supervision by a dietician with a focus on adequate provision of calories (≤30 kcal/kg/day) in order to promote protein sparing and prevent the development of malnutrition.

Ikizler TA, Cuppari L. The 2020 updated KDOQI Clinical Practice Guidelines for nutrition in chronic kidney disease. Blood Purif. 2021;50(4–5):667–71.

235. A. Diet and low-dose statin.

Dietary/lifestyle changes alone are often insufficient to decrease LDL-cholesterol levels to <2.59 mmol/L, particularly in adult kidney transplant recipients with LDL-cholesterol levels of ≤3.36 mmol/L. Therefore, alongside dietary changes, a statin should be prescribed. Statin treatment should be initiated at a low dose and gradually increased until the LDL-cholesterol level reaches a value <2.59 mmol/L.

Kasiske B, Cosio FG, Beto J, et al. Clinical practice guidelines for managing dyslipidemias in kidney transplant patients: a report from the Managing Dyslipidemias in Chronic Kidney Disease Work Group of the National Kidney Foundation Kidney Disease Outcomes Quality Initiative. Am J Transplant. 2004;4(Suppl 7):13–53.

236. B. Haemodialysis.

Ethylene glycol is metabolised in the liver by alcohol dehydrogenase to glycolic acid, glyoxylic acid, and oxalic acid. These cause cytotoxic tubular injury, renal tubular calcium oxalate precipitation, and metabolic acidosis. Glycolic acid and glyoxylic acid produce falsely elevated lactate levels by activating L-lactate oxidase found in blood gas analysers.

Fomepizole and intravenous ethanol both inhibit the action of alcohol dehydrogenase. However, Intravenous ethanol causes reduced consciousness; therefore, fomepizole is used in non-critical cases. Haemodialysis eliminates ethylene glycol faster than haemofiltration. Haemodialysis should be utilized when ethylene glycol levels are >500 mg/L or in the presence of AKI, metabolic acidosis, cardiovascular instability/arrhythmias, or neurological deficits.

In: J Feehally, J Floege, M Tonelli, eds. Comprehensive Clinical Nephrology, 6th edition. St Louis, MO: Elsevier, 2019; Chapters 16–26.

237. E. Tubulointerstitial nephritis.

Individuals with HIV are at risk of both AKI and CKD. Both are associated with significant morbidity and mortality. AKI can result directly from HIV glomerulonephropathies or can be secondary to antiretroviral medications. FSGS is a common HIV glomerulonephropathy but is not associated with temperatures, joint pain, or eosinophilia.

The combination of joint pain, low-grade temperature, eosinophilia, and proteinuria suggests a diagnosis of acute tubulointerstitial nephritis secondary to abacavir. It is uncommon for lamivudine and dolutegravir to have nephrotoxic effects.

Nolin TD, Perazella MA. Introduction to Nephropharmacology for the Clinician: A New CJASN Series. Clin J Am Soc Nephrol. 2018 Jul 6;13(7):1083–4.

238. B. Bendroflumethiazide.

In renal impairment, allopurinol metabolites can accumulate and toxicity results in allopurinol hypersensitivity syndrome (AHS). AHS is rare, but life-threatening, and typically occurs within weeks after allopurinol initiation or with concomitant use of thiazide diuretics. AHS can clinically present with a severe cutaneous adverse reaction (SCAR), drug rash with eosinophilia and systemic symptoms (DRESS), Stevens–Johnson syndrome (SJS), toxic epidermal necrolysis (TEN), hepatitis, vasculitis, acute kidney injury, and eosinophilia. Once a serious hypersensitivity reaction is confirmed, allopurinol should not be reintroduced.

Hande KR, Noone RM, Stone WJ. Severe allopurinol toxicity. Description and guidelines for prevention in patients with renal insufficiency. Am J Med. 1984;76(1):47–56.

Hui M, Carr A, Cameron S, et al. The British Society for Rheumatology guideline for the management of gout. Rheumatology. 2017;56(7):1–20.

239. A. High anion gap acidosis.

Co-administration of paracetamol and flucloxacillin causes high anion gap pyroglutamic metabolic acidosis (PGA). PGA is more likely to occur in individuals with renal or liver dysfunction, sepsis, or malnutrition. PGA occurs because intravenous acetaminophen results in low glutathione and elevated 5-oxoprolinase levels. Flucloxacillin inhibits 5-oxoprolinase to 5-oxoproline (also known as pyroglutamic acid). This leads to elevated levels of pyroglutamic acid, resulting in a high anion gap acidosis.

Treatment is supportive: changing analgesia and switching antibiotics, hydration, and correction of acidosis with sodium bicarbonate.

Emmett M. Acetaminophen toxicity and 5-oxoproline (pyroglutamic acid): a tale of two cycles, one an ATP-depleting futile cycle and the other a useful cycle. Clin J Am Soc Nephrol. 2014;9:191–200.

240. A. Dapaglifozin.

The treatment algorithm for glucose-lowering medication in type 2 diabetes is dependent on the presence or absence of CKD, heart failure, or atherosclerotic cardiovascular disease.

In the presence of CKD or heart failure, SLGT2I are first line if the eGFR is >20 mL/min/1.73 m². Metformin is used when the eGFR is >30 mL/min/1.73 m². Saxagliptin cannot be used in CKD.

Davies MJ, Aroda VR, Collins BS, et al. Management of Hyperglycemia in Type 2 Diabetes, 2022. A Consensus Report by the American Diabetes Association (ADA) and the European Association for the Study of Diabetes (EASD). Diabetes Care. 2022 Nov 1;45(11):275–2786.

241. C. Oxycodone.

Neuropathic pain is common within the diabetic CKD and ESRD population. It is important to optimize glycaemic control and rule out reversible causes, including excessive alcohol consumption, B12 deficiency, and thyroid dysfunction. The first-line therapy is either calcium channel alpha-2-delta ligands (gabapentin/pregabalin) or tricyclic antidepressants. Only after first-line management has been maximally uptitrated, should non-opioid analgesia (paracetamol) be added. Avoid NSAIDs as they can precipitate further renal decline. Subsequent steps include addition and uptitration of an opioid (tramadol, oxycodone, hydromorphone). Pain refractory to pharmacological treatment warrants referral to the pain team. Surgery is not indicated.

Nolin TD, Perazella MA. Introduction to Nephropharmacology for the Clinician: A New CJASN Series. Clin J Am Soc Nephrol. 2018 Jul 6;13(7):1083–4.

Davidson SN, Koncicki H, Brennan FP. Pain in chronic kidney disease: a scoping review. Semin Dial. 2014;27(2):188–204.

242. C. Discuss end-of-life care with the patient and family.

This gentleman shows evidence of multisystem failure and has advanced, progressive, and incurable illnesses, not tolerating dialysis, and with severe left ventricular systolic function leading to increased frailty. Hypotension due to left ventricular systolic dysfunction will not respond to fludrocortisone. Fluids will exacerbate pulmonary oedema, and inotropes would be invasive and not alter the prognosis. Peritoneal dialysis is a valid alternative dialysis treatment, but not in the context of a frail gentleman with intractable low BP secondary to end-stage heart failure.

NHS Improving Quality (2015). End of life care in advanced kidney disease: a framework for implementation. Available from: https://www.england.nhs.uk/improvement-hub/wp-content/uploads/sites/44/2017/11/Advanced-kidney-disease.pdf

Russon L, Mooney A. Palliative and end-of-life care in advanced renal failure. Clin Med (Lond). 2010;10(3):279–81.

243. C. Gabapentin.

Uraemic pruritus is prevalent in 11% of individuals with CKD stages 3–5. Biochemical causes of pruritus, such as hyperphosphataemia, hyperparathyroidism, and poor dialysis adequacy, should be excluded. Topical emollients or moisturizing ointments are the first-line treatments, followed by the introduction of a calcium channel alpha-2-delta ligand (gabapentin/pregabalin).

There is no role for antihistamines, as they do not target the underlying pathophysiology of uraemic pruritus. There are minimal data that γ-linolenic acid (GLA) found in evening primrose oil is beneficial, however, it is not part of the management ladder. Dermatology referral for UVB phototherapy is appropriate after topical and oral management therapies have failed. The phosphate level is not elevated and therefore not the cause of itching.

Manenti L, Tansinda P, Vaglio A. Uraemic pruritus clinical characteristics, pathophysiology and treatment. Drugs. 2009;69(3):251–63.

Mettang T, Kremer AE. Uremic pruritus. Kidney Int. 2015;87:685–91.

244. D. Subcutaneous midazolam, alfentanil, and hyoscine butylbromide PRN.

PRN subcutaneous medications are used to manage intermittent symptoms, whereas persistent symptoms require medicine delivery via a syringe driver. Midazolam and alfentanil are used in the management of intermittent symptoms of agitation and breathlessness respectively. Hyoscine butylbromide is used in the management of respiratory tract secretions. Haloperidol and levomepromazine are used for nausea and vomiting.

NHS Lothian (2014). Renal palliative care: last days of life. Available from: https://www.palliativecare ggc.org.uk/wp-content/uploads/2015/08/RenalLastDays-nov-2013.pdf

245. D. Patiromer.

Initial management of moderate hyperkalaemia (6.0–6.4 mmol/L) is a low-potassium diet, medication review (ACE inhibitors, ARBs, mineralocorticoid receptor agonists, beta-blockers), and correction of metabolic acidosis (if the bicarbonate level is <22 mmol/L).

Patiromer is a gut potassium binder and increases the excretion of potassium in faeces. It is a slow-acting treatment for hyperkalaemia and is used in individuals with persistent hyperkalaemia (6.0 mmol/L) and CKD stages 3b to 5 or heart failure.

National Institute for Health and Care Excellence (2020). Patiromer for treating hyperkalaemia. Technology appraisal guidance [TA623]. Available from: https://www.nice.org.uk/guidance/ta623/chapter/1-Recommendations

Take-Home Messages

1. Malnutrition results from multiple mechanisms, leading to protein–energy wasting states in individuals requiring RRT.
2. The Subjective Global Assessment is the gold standard for the evaluation of nutritional status in the dialysis population.
3. Protein requirements in people with AKI are influenced by the individual's catabolic state and type of RRT.
4. Low/very low-protein diets in people with CKD stages 3 and 4 should be implemented, alongside adequate provision of calories to prevent malnutrition.
5. Dietary changes and a low-dose statin should be the first approach to treat hyperlipidaemia In adult kidney transplant recipients.
6. Haemodialysis/haemofiltration is needed to eliminate ethylene glycol and metabolites in severe ethylene glycol toxicity.
7. Abacavir is a common antiretroviral drug in the treatment of HIV and can cause tubulointerstitial nephritis.
8. AHS is a rare, but life-threatening, complication of use of allopurinol in individuals with CKD. AHS occurs either after commencing allopurinol or with concomitant use of thiazide diuretics.
9. High-risk individuals need to be monitored closely during co-administration of intravenous paracetamol and flucloxacillin for the development of pyroglutamic metabolic acidosis.
10. The type 2 diabetes management algorithm has a treatment arm for individuals with CKD, starting with SLGT2i and GLP-1 RA.
11. The analgesic pain ladder for individuals with CKD starts with commencing and uptitrating gabapentin/pregabalin or tricyclic antidepressants. Non-opioid analgesia is subsequently added, followed by the addition of opioids.
12. It is imperative to have an advanced care plan for individuals with advanced, progressive, incurable illnesses and to have clear, open discussions with the patient and their family.
13. Management of uraemic pruritus initially involves topical emollients, followed by low-dose gabapentin.
14. While providing palliative care therapy, intermittent symptoms should be managed with PRN medications, whereas persistent symptoms should be managed with a syringe driver.
15. Patiromer is a potassium binder used in the management of moderate hyperkalaemia.

INDEX

For the benefit of digital users, indexed terms that span two pages (e.g., 52–53) may, on occasion, appear on only one of those pages

Tables and figures are indicated by *t* and *f* following the page number